THE EYEBROW

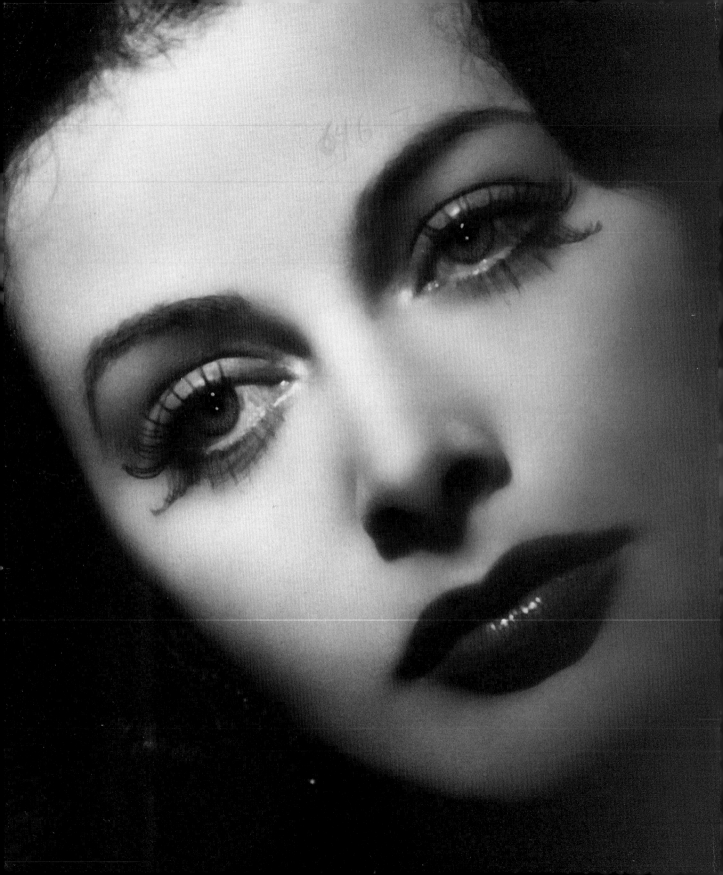

THE EYEBROW

Robyn Cosio with Cynthia Robins

ReganBooks
An Imprint of HarperCollins*Publishers*

Photography credits appear on page 187, which constitutes an extention of this copyright page.

HarperCollins books may be purchased for educational, business, or sales promotional use. For information please write: Special Markets Department, HarperCollins Publishers Inc., 10 East 53rd Street, New York, NY 10022.

FIRST EDITION

Designed by Jeannette Jacobs

Printed on acid-free paper

Library of Congress Cataloging-in-Publication Data has been applied for.

ISBN 0-06-039326-2

00 01 02 03 04 RRD 10 9 8 7 6 5 4 3 2 1

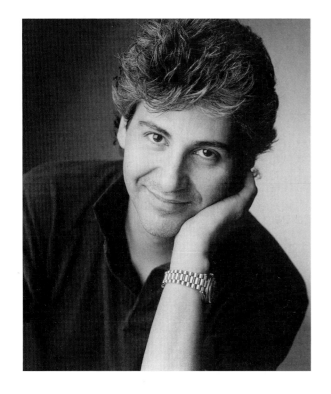

For my darling husband, Armando, and his incredible

sense of beauty. He taught me everything I know.

His memory will be engraved in my heart forever.

MARCH 31, 1946–SEPTEMBER 22, 1990

CONTENTS

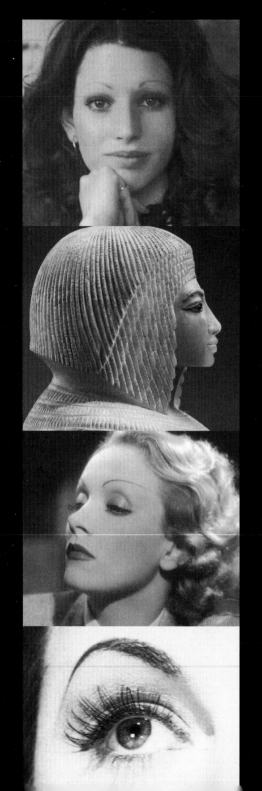

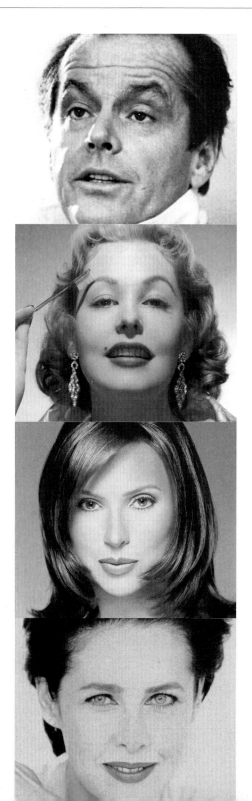

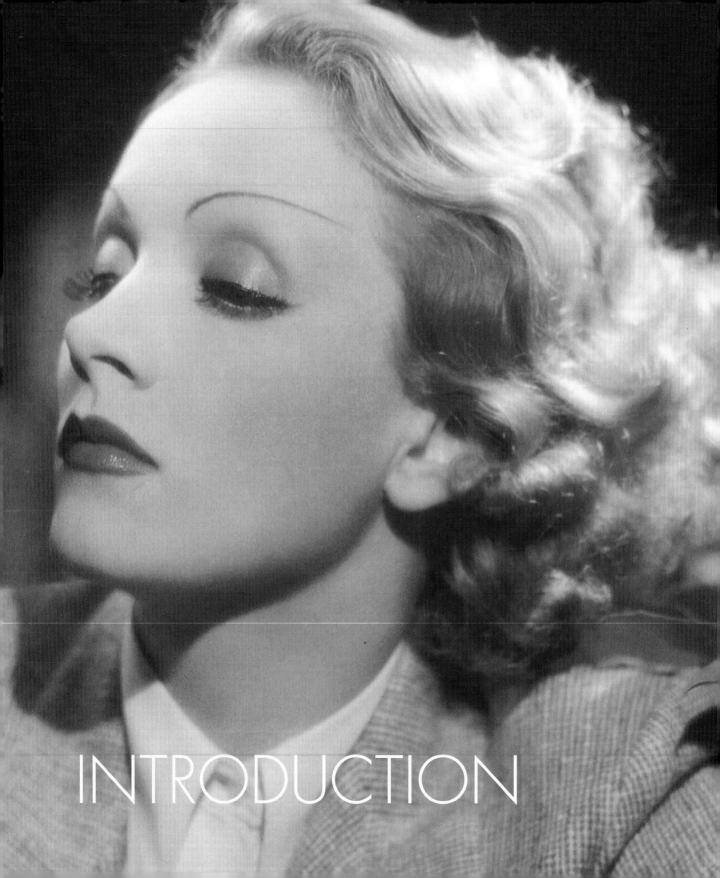

INTRODUCTION

As far back as I can remember, I have been attracted to the glamour of classic beauty. I've always loved those 1940s films in which everything looked so polished, so finished. Women and men looked beautiful from head to toe. From makeup to hair to clothes, shoes, purses, and jewelry—classic style meant less is more. I bring this love of simplicity to my work with eyebrows, creating a perfect, timeless arch that allows a woman's natural beauty to shine through.

There is a certain allure to finding a woman's beauty hidden in her brows. When a woman sits in my chair with her face tilted toward me, her expression filled with hope (or doubt, if she's a first-timer), I know exactly what I'm going to do. I can see her perfect brows—how they will look when I'm finished, how much more beautiful they will be, even a month later. When a woman sits in my chair, I know that despite the condition of her brows—overtweezed, having an unfortunate hole, or never touched at all—I will be able to create the right brows for her.

What other calling allows you to give women an instant "face lift" that will elevate their spirits as well as widen and enlarge their eyes? The eyebrow is the basic framework of the face. Without a groomed brow that is perfect for the face it sits on, a woman's face and her complementary makeup are only half finished. Mona Lisa without her smile. Jackie O. without her dark glasses. Audrey Hepburn without her Fabulous Fifties winged eyebrows.

Marlene Dietrich

Like most girls, I learned my first beauty lessons from watching my mom. She was the best of moms. She looked like Donna Reed. She was a serious homemaker and was always perfectly groomed. I remember when she used to get her lipsticks from the Avon Lady: tiny samples in shiny gold tubes. She'd line them up in a transparent case on her vanity in the bathroom, and I'd go in and smell them. To me, they were romantic and beautiful.

One of my first recollections of beauty? Those lipsticks and my mother, fresh from her bath, standing nude in the bathroom in a fine cloud of Heaven Scent talcum powder. With a huge puff, she'd fluff it on. What struck me then and stays with me now is that memorable scent and how precise those lipsticks looked, standing all in a row . . . and what promise of glamour and undiscovered romance they held.

My dad was an electrician, but what he really was was an artist. He originally started out as a dancer in New York, but with a wife and a child on the way, he needed a job. He came to California to work. My parents settled in Sherman Oaks, in the San Fernando Valley when it was just orange groves and cow pastures.

As I grew into my teens, my mother kept me from exploring my beauty. Oh no, she told me. You can't wear makeup until you're sixteen. Of course, I was piling it on at school. I would "borrow" her eye makeup and foundation (which by the way was at least four shades darker than my pale skin) and slather it on. Sometimes I do makeup for the

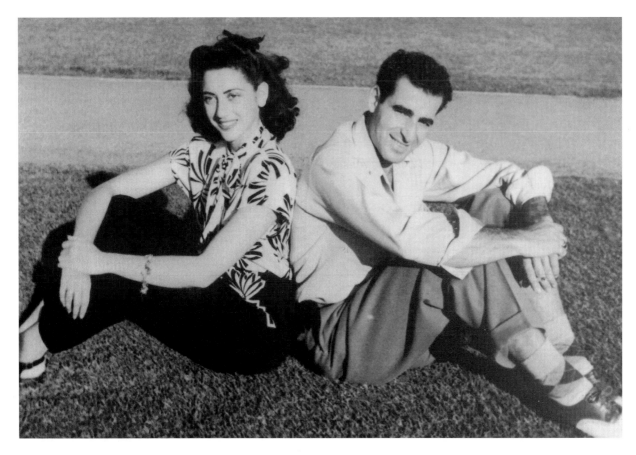

My parents in the late 1940s. As you can see, I come from a family of eyebrows.

dancers of the American Ballet Theatre so they can be seen by the people in the last row. I have to laugh, because that's how I looked in broad daylight in the 1960s.

I have very curly hair, and it was a disaster area—long and out of control—when I was a teenager. So were my eyebrows. I had what is known as the dreaded "unibrow," and my mother forbade me from doing anything about it. But not for long.

Talk about being in the right place at the right time! The 1960s were Rebellion City and I moved right on in. I created a look for myself that was totally up-to-the-minute, inventing myself as I went along. At night, I'd sleep with my hair wrapped around beer cans to straighten it, and I'd plop on two falls of fake hair the next day to complete the effect. I wore two sets of false lashes on both my upper and lower eyelids—they looked like caterpillars on my sink when I took them off—white lips, heavy black eyeliner . . . and no eyebrows. I shaved them off and then painstakingly drew them back on, one by one, with a pencil. Sophia Loren was in vogue then. And her brows were a collection of teensy, perpendicular lines, sketched on to cover her wonderful brow bone. My mother was horrified. It was not the image she had plotted for her older daughter. But I was using myself as an ongoing art project. A living canvas.

In the 1960s in L.A., rock-and-roll was king. Skinny little groupie girls hung out on Sunset Boulevard trying to meet rock stars. Some even got to be famous. There were Frank Zappa's GTOs— Girls Together Only—and the other fearless females like me. I was an official go-go dancer at the Whiskey, the hottest place on the Sunset Strip, where all the rockers and their women hung out.

I'd dance the night away and then stay up in Laurel Canyon with rockers like Jim Morrison, Janis Joplin, and Jimi Hendrix. We girls traipsed around in miniskirts, fishnet stockings, towering platform shoes, skimpy halter tops, bell bottoms, and little blue specs; wore flowers and beads in our hair; and were generally tripping out on life. We were real style-setters, with our long, center-parted hair, our tie-dyes and fringes, and our lithe little bodies. Joni Mitchell laid a name on us: The Ladies of the Canyon.

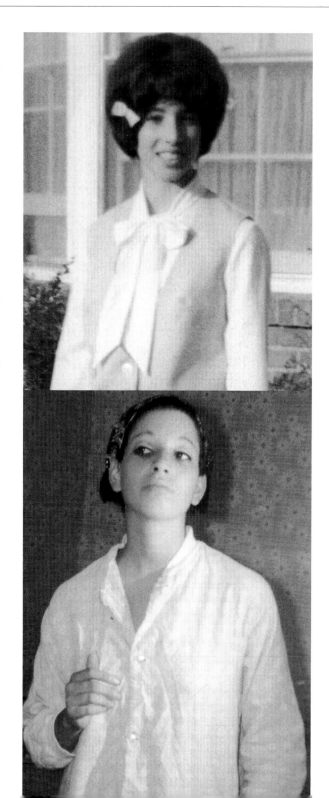

TOP: *Here I am at fourteen, looking like a geek, the last time I allowed my mother to dress me.*
BOTTOM: *By fifteen I was planning my escape.*

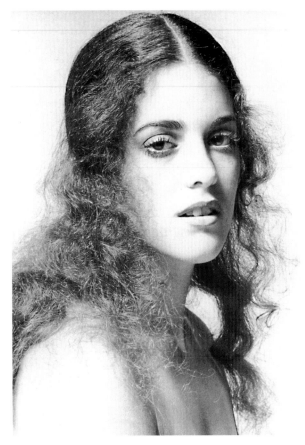

My sister, Wendy, was the all-natural hippie, while my motto was, the more makeup the better.

My mother had no idea what I was doing, personally or even fashionwise. I ran away from home to live with the people I considered the most visionary in town. The artist in me knew that somewhere inside this very young, very impres-

Around 1970, I drew in eyebrows above my actual eyebrows.

sionable girl-woman was a creative soul just waiting to get out. Our group of decorative girls was way ahead of everybody else. The avant-garde. While the totally natural, no-makeup look was spreading through the hippie movement, our physical beauty was anything but natural. We loved cosmetics.

My look was nothing I could (or even wanted to) accomplish in an instant. Like a matador suiting up for an important corrida, I would spend at least three hours a night on my makeup, with such obsession that if I made one mistake, if one false eyelash was out of place, I'd wash it all off and start from

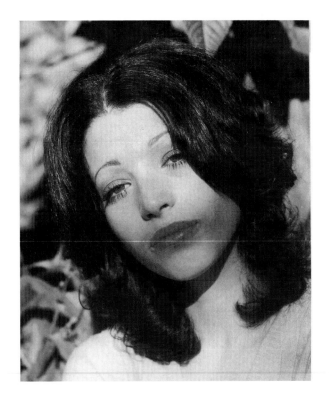

scratch. Today, I don't have the patience or the time . . . and neither do you.

Looking back at my days as a Lady of the Canyon living my mother's worst nightmare, I wish I would have done some things differently, but then I wouldn't be where I am now. Had I stayed the polite little girl my mother preferred, I never would have met Armando Cosio when I was seventeen. He was twenty-four at the time, older and wiser than me, and it was he who started me on the path I follow today.

The day I met Armando in 1967, my life changed forever. I fell in love instantly. I thought he was an incredibly handsome man. He had hypnotic eyes, a charismatic personality, and a patient way about him. He had a natural mystery to him that made him even more exciting, not just to me, but to everyone who met him.

When I met Armando, he was just getting out of beauty school. In the next few years, his reputation as a hair stylist grew and he became quite famous. His client list was heavy with the names of the rich and famous, mostly movie stars. When he opened his own shop, he hired me to be his receptionist. One of the perks of the job was that I got to hang out and watch. When Armando added makeup to his hairdressing skills, he became much in demand for photo shoots and magazine layouts. He worked for the great glamour photographers of the age: Helmut Newton, Richard Avedon, Victor Skrebneski, Francesco Scavullo, Irving Penn. He gave Raquel

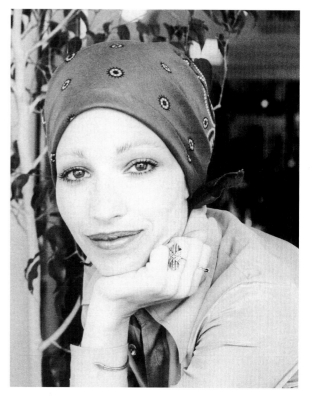

I shaved off my eyebrows and drew them in with a No. 2 lead pencil, line by line, à la Sophia Loren.

Welch her first short hair. He cut and blonded Olivia Newton John's hair, held it back with a terry headband, and helped her "Get Physical." He styled Linda Evans's hair through her *Dynasty* years.

In the beauty industry, you can't stay a receptionist for long if you want to be successful. Forget about famous; I just wanted to try my wings. My first bona fide, hands-on job in the beauty industry? I became a manicurist at Carrie White's, *the* Beverly Hills buff-and-puff parlor of the early '70s. When I

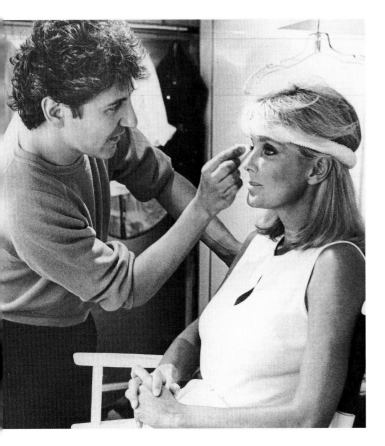

Armando and Linda Evans.

Xavier Salon at Fifty-seventh Street and Fifth Avenue, the best salon in New York, where I sold myself as a makeup artist by doing a simple makeup on one of their shampoo girls. They asked me to start right away. I panicked. I made up an excuse: I had a shoot for a commercial and would be back in two weeks. I flew home and "studied" with Armando. He gave me a full makeup kit and taught me everything I needed in the way of technique. I returned to New York, armed and ready to start the next phase of my life as a makeup artist.

My parents had sent me to art school when I was ten. I knew about what artists call "chiaroscuro"—that light colors make things stick out and dark colors make them recede. As Armando was teaching me, my art school training (and some of my father's artistic leanings) came back to me. But I had never worked on a three-dimensional canvas before. Armando gave me the best advice possible: "Just pretend it's your own face."

In New York I was young, raw, ambitious, and, as I look back now, fearless. (As in, what you don't know can't hurt you.) I knew no one. I didn't have a crew . . . or a clue, for that matter. As green as I was, I knew instinctively that I was going in the right direction.

There are always beginning makeup artists whose main ambition is to eventually get noticed by a large cosmetics company. They wanted to work their way up from line girl at Bloomingdale's to a

wasn't painting nails, I was teaching clients like Julie Christie and Betsy Bloomingdale how to disco.

I was getting bored with manicuring nails, so I danced myself right out of Beverly Hills. In 1976 I followed a boyfriend to New York City, and then I did what I always did when I needed advice: I called Armando—this time from a phone booth on Fifth Avenue—and said, "What should I do now?"

"Do makeup," he said. "You're good at it."

Sometimes things happen when you need them to. I hung up the phone and walked over to the

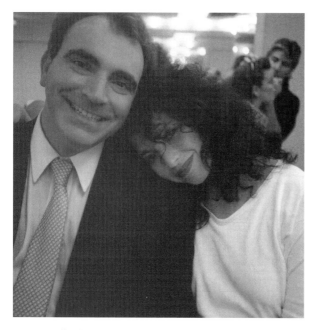

Louis Dell'Olio and I at one of my first jobs designing makeup for the Anne Klein collection.

traveling trainer for a large cosmetics company. That was the last thing I wanted to do. What I envisioned: my name in the cover credits of a well-known fashion magazine, my "faces" smiling out from the pages of a luxury catalog, my "girls" striding down a catwalk. I decided that I was designed for the glamorous life. Traveling to exotic locations, working with beautiful models and topflight photographers—that's what I wanted for myself. (Looking back on it now, it was exactly the life that Armando had.)

Maybe I was impatient, or maybe I was just a fast learner, but achieving my dream was a very

When I wasn't working, I spent all my time at Studio 54.

efficient process. I was not afraid of hard work, and, from experience, I realized that the worst thing anyone could say was no, and that, if I was confident enough, they'd probably say, "Yes!"

My friends have always said: "Robyn starts from the top, never from the bottom." I simply jumped into the world I wanted. I was willing to work hard, to go just about anywhere to build up my portfolio. When I was a beginner, I would do the makeup for test shots for new models and journeymen photographers. I would go anywhere, any time, and for just about anyone. I would work until three in the morning in a blizzard and take the subway home. It didn't matter, just as long as I got to do makeup.

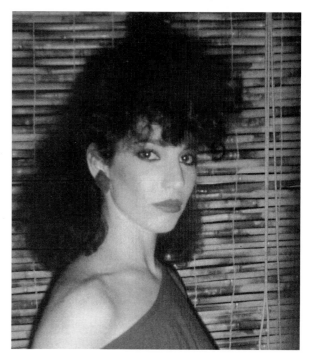

My first editorial job was in 1976 for *Mademoiselle.* Each night before the shoots, I would call Armando in Los Angeles and he would coach me and walk me through any problems. But there never really were any—he had taught me well. All I knew was that I was having the best time of my life, doing what I loved. And starting to make money at it. What could be better?

My big break came when I did my very first runway makeup for the hot team of Louis Dell'Olio and Donna Karan, who were codesigning the Anne Klein fashion line. Next came shows for Claude Montana, Bill Blass, Stephen Burrows, Perry Ellis, Oscar de la Renta, and many other New York design stars. I worked for little money until I established my reputation and put my "book" together.

After I had been a makeup artist for a few years, I began to realize that when a woman sat in my chair with a clean face, my eyes would go directly to her brows, and I'd think to myself, "Boy, is *that* a mess. Before I start the makeup, I have to clean this up." But I'm a pretty honest person, and there were times when I'd tell the client what I thought. If she asked me, "Do you like the shape?" I'd answer, "What shape?" Women laughed at my frankness, leaned back, and let me tweeze away on them before I even started with paint and powder.

I spent eight years in New York. Then Armando decided he missed me and wanted me home. We had grown closer over the years, and little by little, he fell in love with me. I had *always* been in love with him.

When I finally moved back to Los Angeles to live with Armando, I put away my makeup brushes and paints and powders and took a break from beauty.

Donna Karan asked me to be her West Coast rep for her first solo collection. "You're the perfect DK woman," she told me. I worked with her for six months and realized that I didn't understand fabric very well. Besides, I was restless and needed another canvas. The outdoors. I decided to become a landscape artist. Just as with my first job as a makeup artist, I didn't know anything about that, either. I bought a garden book about the flora of the West, read it from cover to cover, and traded fringey lashes and lip gloss for ground cover and perennials.

Meanwhile, my wildest dream had come true. My best friend had fallen in love with me. Armando became all things to me: not only my best friend, but my teacher, my guide, my lover, and then, my husband. I couldn't have asked for anything better. For the first time in my life, I felt safe. We traveled the world on his assignments; we vacationed in storybook places. We had homes in Santa Fe and Los Angeles. We were surrounded by a circle of talented and loving friends. Nothing could touch us.

Or so we thought. Our carefully constructed idyll shattered in an instant when we discovered that Armando had contracted the AIDS virus. It was devastating news.

Little did we know what lay ahead for us. Together, we started on a journey that was so sad and immensely painful that there was nowhere to go but down. My heart and my life were disintegrating at the same rate as Armando's immune system. Watching Armando through this debilitating illness destroyed my soul.

Through it all, Armando never complained. I was always in awe of him and, through his sickness, even more so. No one could have been more beautiful, inside and out. People choose to die in many ways. Some want to be alone and cut themselves off from their loved ones. Others leave life as they have lived it—graciously and lovingly.

I knew that I needed and wanted to complete our final chapter together, so we were married on April 22, 1988, nearly two and a half years before he passed away. Until the day I die, I will cherish this very special and unique man. There will never be another Armando.

As I look back on it now, I try so hard to put the devastation of our experience into perspective and focus on the positive. Our life together was filled with friends and family, adventure and affection. For a while, before the sickness took its toll, we were able to travel and spent a glorious time in Hawaii. Little did I know that it would be our last trip.

The last two or three months of his life were the most difficult to deal with. I was in total denial that I was losing this man. I was with him constantly. But Armando and my friends insisted that I get out of the house. And I needed to. I would be no good to Armando if I were too exhausted and burned out. A friend suggested that maybe I'd want to go back to

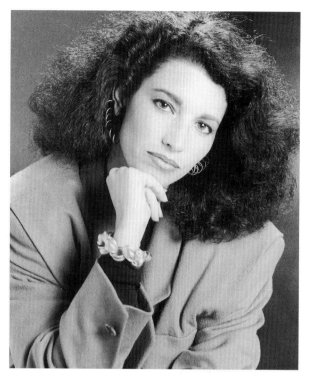

My eyebrows grew back just in time for the Eighties.

doing makeup a couple of days a week. The owner of the Umberto Salon in Beverly Hills had known Armando's reputation and hired me for two days a week. Umberto's manager, Babette, offered to teach me how to wax eyebrows. My initial reaction was, "*Eeeuuwww.* I don't want to do that. I'm a makeup artist!" Some snob I was. But she said, "It's a good way to pick up some easy money. It's fast, and you can make ten dollars a set." That was in 1990.

I'll never forget my first client, the first real person I ever touched with hot wax. She was a very fussy Frenchwoman, probably in her seventies, a grande

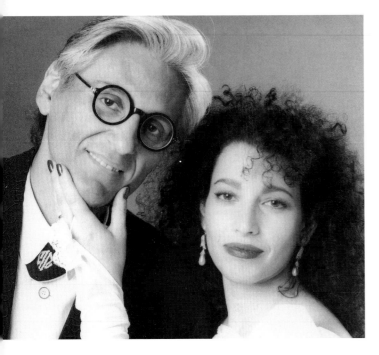

Armando and I at our wedding.

I have become very proficient at what I do. It takes me exactly four minutes to wax a set of eyebrows. I can probably work on five clients within the space of a half hour. When I am in New York one week a month, I am booked so tightly that I often do forty to fifty sets of brows in a day.

I do not sugarcoat my criticism of a client's at-home tweezing transgressions. I can always tell when they've been at their brows or had someone else do them. Nor do I care if the current trend dictates that brows be narrowed, trimmed, or dyed—or that they resemble an untamed pile of brush. Instead, I insist that each pair of brows I work on be appropriate for the face to which they're attached.

A session with me begins the same way with each client. First I survey what I need to do, then I tell them, "Turn your head toward me," and brush their brow hairs toward the outer hairline. I will place honey-scented hot wax on the superfluous hairs I call "the negative"—hairs that obscure the line I want both under and above the true brow. Before the wax has time to cool, I place a rectangle of clean, natural muslin on the wax, tamp it down, and pull, very suddenly, against the direction the hairs grow. Most of my clients are so used to this, they hardly flinch, although there is just a second of discomfort. But the result!

The perfect brow is not an instant fix. It is a cumulative process. Very few of my clients walk away with what I imagine as perfection. I enlist their help. I tell them that it's just like letting bangs grow out.

dame—and a tiny terror. She was extremely particular and very, very touchy. As I lifted the orange stick loaded with hot wax up and over her body, a blob fell onto her collar, her starched, embroidered white collar on a blouse that I knew she was going to wear to lunch at the Bistro Garden. She was furious. The salon paid for her blouse.

I could have quit on the spot, but that is not my nature. I kept at it, gaining speed and skill. I moved to another salon, and my reputation grew. I started working on high-profile women in the entertainment business: the late Dawn Steel, one of the first female studio heads; Amy Pascal, now chairman of Columbia Studios; and lots of directors, producers, and actresses.

They've got to be patient. So many of them have been doing their brows themselves or have allowed people work on them who perhaps have made mistakes. They've taken out too many hairs or too many of the *wrong* hairs. Clients come to me with what has become a brow reclamation project.

Most of my clients have been coming to me for years. If they miss an appointment for some reason, they are very apologetic about it. And sometimes a client feels the need to confess: "Gee, Robyn, I haven't touched my brows since the last time I saw you. Just a few straight down the middle." I definitely have them trained. They know I won't be happy if I see they've been picking away at them. It's called beauty by intimidation. And it works.

When I look at a "virgin" brow, one that I have not worked on before, I can see in my mind's eye the perfect shape hidden under all of those stray hairs. It may be a skill born of experience—I've made up thousands of faces over the past twenty-three years—but I have the instinct to know what is right for the face in front of me.

Sometimes a brand-new client will come to me with a photograph of her ideal brow and say, "I want *those*!" when she has only five hairs to work with. It is my job to be honest with her and tell her what I can do. And I am very blunt when I need to be. Either they get it or they don't. And sometimes, they're in shock because I tell them the truth.

Luckily for me, these women—movie stars, trophy wives, models, executives, ballerinas, teenagers, soccer moms, doctors, attorneys, coeds, debutantes, and secretaries—trust me. Women are able to put their faces in my hands, their brows under my black and silver tweezers, and know that they will, with my help and guidance, turn out perfectly.

I'd like to share a little story with you. One day at the Peter Coppola Salon, one of my regular clients, a peppery, darkly beautiful book editor and publisher named Judith Regan, sat in my chair, listened to some of my stories, and announced, "Robyn, *you* should write a book. Not everyone has the chance to sit in your chair, and you know so much. Share it with people."

So, in the following pages, you're going to learn everything you ever thought you'd want to know about the eyebrow. We're going to look at the eyebrow through history; we'll learn the secrets of the world's most beautiful women, from Cleopatra and Queen Elizabeth I to Jean Harlow, Elizabeth Taylor, Jean Shrimpton, and Cindy Crawford. And I'll show you step by step how to divine, design, and do your own eyebrows.

In the new millennium, the well-groomed modern woman should look back to the simplest principles of glamour that Hollywood's greatest movie queens—such as Gene Tierney, Rita Hayworth, Ava Gardner, and Audrey Hepburn—understood. It's not glitter eye shadow, black eyeliner, and a foundation applied with a trowel that makes a woman beautiful. It is—and make this your beauty mantra—a gorgeous mouth, clear, beautiful skin, great hair, and stunning eyebrows.

THE
EYEBROW
THROUGH
HISTORY

When Mother Nature created the eyebrow, little did she ever suspect that it would become the object of so much décor. That it could be arched elegantly; tweezed into oblivion; dyed beyond recognition; pierced and garnished with rings, barbells, spikes, and safety pins, or left completely to fend for itself.

As long as human beings have been on Earth, they have indulged in some kind of makeup ritual. Since before recorded time, the eyebrow has played a role in the decoration of a face. Even in ages where brows were left to wander as they chose, they made some kind of fashion or cultural statement.

Information about eyebrow modification and beautification of women from ancient to modern times has come in all forms. Archaeologists digging into the tombs of ancient Crete, Egypt, Greece, and Rome discovered decorative cosmetic boxes complete with miniature tools and pots of pigment. Burial paintings, frescoes, urns, and busts were the portraits that recorded the prevailing fashion in both clothing and face painting. In later societies, poets,

Both men and women in the Egyptian royal court painted their eyes and eyebrows with kohl and with crushed minerals such as powdered green malachite. Statues and busts from the ancient periods found in tombs show evidence of heavy cosmetics use and graphically drawn eyebrows. Canopic jar lid (detail), Dynasty XVIII, ca. 1340–1330 B.C.E., Princess Meryetaten from tomb of Queen Teye, Thebes; The Metropolitan Museum of Art, The Theodore M. Davis Collection, Bequest of Theodore M. Davis, 1915.

historians, monks, and priests kept records of the fashions of the times, although in the Middle Ages, the Church scribes tended to look askance at any kind of artifice as the mark of the Devil. Still later, when men and women of quality and means began traveling the world, their diaries produced vivid descriptions of the fashions of the day in exotic, faraway societies.

Advice books on beauty probably date from Georgian England, where men—doctors and charlatans alike—and impoverished noblewomen wrote their instructions into books and pamphlets in an attempt to remain out of the poorhouse. In the Victorian and Edwardian periods in both the United States and England, ladies' magazines printed recipes for concoct-at-home cosmetics—particularly skin creams, eau de cologne, soap, and hair dye. Fashion magazines, starting with *Vogue* more than a hundred years ago, chronicled the styles of the day and doled out makeup tips, advice, and advertisements for mass-marketed cosmetics.

In each period, the eyebrow, the chief indicator of emotion and expression on the face, has spoken louder than any word that has issued from the lips. Governed by tiny muscles in the forehead, eyebrows can't help what they say. They arch when they want to show surprise, they knit together with concern, they beetle when they are concerned, and they can operate independently from one another in expressions of anger, irony, or joy. Much of the time their human owners have little control over them. So it

1

surprises no one that eyebrow decoration throughout the ages has been an attempt to corral, control, highlight, and emphasize those independent critters whose job it is to frame the face.

Makeup, as a mark of civilization, began in prehistoric times. Cosmetics were tribal codes and the signature of the shaman, who used animal grease mixed with ashes and colored with plant dyes to differentiate himself from the rest of the tribe, particularly during rituals meant to protect the clan. The first makeups were berry stains and plant pigments, ashes, or minerals pounded into powder, mixed with bear grease, and smeared onto faces and bodies in bold patterns.

For the earliest literate civilizations that kept track of daily life on tablets and scrolls, dating to five thousand years before the birth of Christ, there are records of how men and women used makeup and where they put it. It wasn't until the rise of the ancient peoples of the Etruscan, Egyptian, Sumerian, and Persian civilizations that man used his eyebrows for any other reasons than to protect his eyes from dust and dirt and the cruel and blinding rays of the sun.

THE EGYPTIANS

It is the Egyptians who have had the longest-running influence on the eyebrow as decoration throughout the centuries. Certainly they were one of the first societies to decorate eyes and brows in elaborate and graphic manners. It is a style icon that has lasted thousands of years.

The Egyptians left evidence of their vanity in the hieroglyphics on tomb walls, but also in the ebony, wood, and ivory cosmetic boxes they buried with their mummified royalty and gentry (along with personal slaves, household items, clothing, and jewelry) to ease their way into their new home in the Underworld.

When British and American adventurers and archaeologists discovered and pillaged the ancient tombs of the Egyptian pharaohs at the end of the nineteenth century and into the 1920s, they unearthed colorful busts and sarcophagus paintings of kings and their famous queens. The glamour portraits of the age, they showed evidence of the use of cosmetics, with darkened brows and maquillaged eyes decorated with green and black paint. The famous head of Nefertiti that resides today in a German museum is a study in careful artifice. Nefertiti was definitely a cosmetics queen. The wife of Akhenaten and queen of Egypt, Nefertiti lived 1,300 years before Christ. She had sloe eyes and large, shapely black brows that went clear to her nose but did not meet. She is considered one of the great beauties of all time.

The ancient Egyptians used antimony powder to blacken their brows and huge black lines of kohl made of galena (black lead) to shape eyelids into wings. All Egyptians of any age, sex, or class decorated their faces. Fashion of the day decreed that the natural brow be shaved off and a new, perfect one be painted on in its place. Both men and women wore the grossly exaggerated eye. Cleopatra either shaved or tweezed her brows (there are hieroglyphics of her contemporaries at their toilette, using tweezers to eliminate their brows) and painted on their replacements. Her upper lids were deep blackish blue and her lower lids were bright green. When archaeologists opened the great tombs of Egypt, they found eye paint made of powdered green malachite in decorative boxes buried with their owners.

Kohl was the most important cosmetic in Egypt. It was made by grinding minerals such as powdered antimony, black manganese oxide, galena (black lead), black oxide of copper, iron oxide, and malachite together with burned almonds and brown ocher. Kohl was kept in pots and then scooped out with a miniature scuttle made of ivory, wood, or gold, into a separate mixing dish, where it was moistened with saliva and applied to the brow or eye with a special kohl stick. Not only were the painted brows decorative and stylish, they were like ancient sunglasses, protecting the eye from the brutal Saharan sun.

The influence of the dramatic Egyptian brow and eye has cropped up through the decades, particularly on the women of other ages, other times, who painted à la Egypt: The ballerinas of the 1920s from the Ballets Russes in Paris, whose heavily made-up eyes were Cleopatraesque; the silent film vamps like Theda Bara, Pola Negri, and Nita Naldi, who kohled

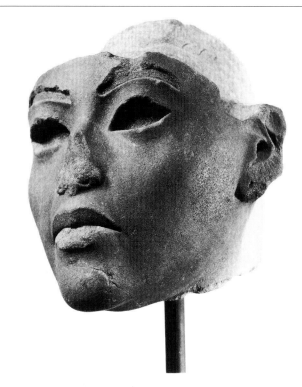

Head of King Akhenaten, Dynasty XVIII, ca. 1363–1347 B.C.E., The Metropolitan Museum of Art, Rogers Fund, 1911.

their eyes, coated their lids with dark shadow, and emphasized their brows with dark pencil; and the millions of women in the mid-1960s who, after they saw Elizabeth Taylor in the film *Cleopatra,* colored their brows with a heavy hand and a lot of black pencil, painted their lids with turquoise shadow, and emphasized their eyes with black liner that took off toward their hairlines on furious wings.

THE ANCIENTS OF THE MEDITERRANEAN

Near Egypt were the civilizations of Crete, Persia, Etruria, Assyria, and Sumeria, all of which decorated faces and eyebrows. Cretan frescoes, dating to 2,500 years ago, show women with doe eyes, dark black eyebrows that are idealized in shape and designed into a thin but definite line. The Etruscans considered wide-set eyes a mark of ravishing beauty. They made up their faces heavily, and arched and emphasized their brows.

The Sumerians stroked a thick mixture of galena and lampblack dissolved in animal fat on their brows. A shell-shaped cosmetics pot made of malachite and gold equipped with a miniature cosmetics spoon and a tiny pair of tweezers was found in a Sumerian tomb. In Persia, after the reign of the Medes, kings went into battle with their cosmetics cases, which were fitted with kohl and tweezers. And the Assyrians, both men and women, blackened their brows and eyelashes with antimony, a brittle, silver-white metal.

THE GREEKS

Unlike the Egyptian civilization, in which women of high birth and breeding were a pretty independent lot, the women of ancient Greece were looked upon as chattel. Properly married women and their daughters did not paint. In the Greek society, where the male ideal fostered love between men, women were shunted aside as keepers of the home and hearth. The Greeks were obsessed with female purity. It was fairly easy to tell the difference between a proper Greek woman and a courtesan; it was on their faces. Prostitutes painted. A writer of the time duly recorded the toilette of a courtesan: "A black coating touched up her eyebrows, and the edges of her eyelids were drawn with a brush dipped in incense black." It was probably the beginning of the physical schism between nice girls and bad girls.

An eyebrow that marched in a single line from one edge of the right eye, over the nose, to the edge of the left eye (known in contemporary times as the "unibrow") was prized as a sign of intelligence and great beauty in women. If a woman was not blessed with one very large and very thick eyebrow, she was allowed to close the gap between her eyes with black paint made of kohl or lampblack. Or she simply put on false eyebrows.

THE ROMANS

The Roman woman had much more freedom and power than her Greek sister. She and her husband lived separate lives in a society that had become corrupted by luxury. With long, lazy, sumptuous dinners and entertainments to give, Roman women were cognizant of style and competitive in their fashions, jewels, and cosmetic rituals. They heaped on the artifice and ostentation. They dyed their hair blond or wore wigs, lightened their faces, and during their bathing rituals, perfumed their hair and eyebrows with essential oils of bergamot and mink. Where nature had blessed them with natural assets, they augmented them with paint, wigs, and artificial eyebrows. The poet Ovid allowed in "The Art of Love" that women's "eyebrows can be made of fur."

A woman was expected to spend hours at her toilette, having her slaves dress her hair into curls and braids, often adding hairpieces in the shape of poufs and bangs. The Roman dramatist Plautus wrote that women without makeup were like food without salt.

The famous poets and writers of the day used their compositions to guide and comment on the beauty rituals of the Roman female. As in Greece, the unibrow look was the reigning fashion, and Ovid duly recorded this instruction: "You have the art to fill in the space between your eyebrows." Lucian, a Greek satirist born in Syria but writing in Rome, referred in "The Lady's Toilet" to "boxes [that] contain only things she would not want any-

The Roman woman loved cosmetics and artifice, but allowed her eyebrows to flourish in all of their luxuriant glory. The J. Paul Getty Museum, Malibu, California, attributed to the Isidora Master, Fayum Mummy Portrait of a Woman *(detail), about 100–125 A.D., encaustic gilt on a wooden panel wrapped in linen, 13 ¼ by 6 ¾ inches.*

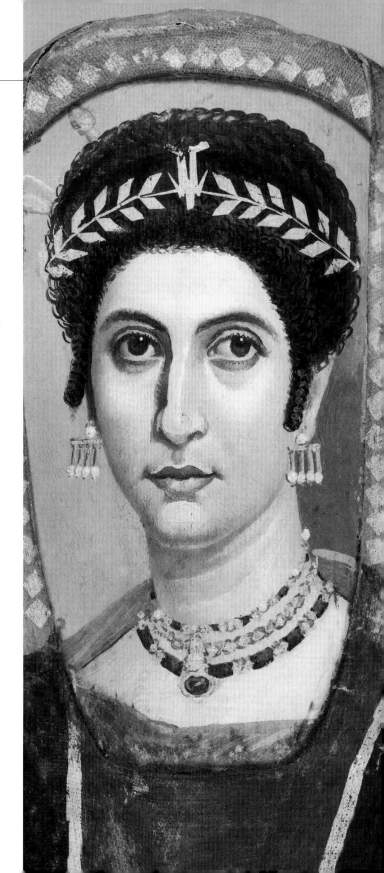

one to see. In one are teeth . . . in another eyelashes and eyebrows and the means of restoring faded beauty." The satirist Petronius, writing in the first century A.D., spoke of a woman using false brows:

> Taking care her eyebrows to be
> Not apart, not mingled, either
> But as hers are, stol'n together
> Met by stealth, yet leaning too
> O'en the eyes their darkest hue.

Both Roman men and women had elaborate cosmetic rituals. The emperor Nero and his wife, Poppaea, used cosmetics. Her beauty ritual was quite complicated and labor intensive. She required a different female slave for each task, and woe to that slave girl who forgot to bring her paints or her box of false brows on time. Like other highborn Roman women of the time, Poppaea would start her countdown to beauty in a bath of asses' milk, and then cover her face with a white, lead-based chalk or a lead paste called "ceruse," which was probably the beginning of a centuries-long addiction to a corrosive and toxic substance that ravaged complexions and caused numerous cosmetic-related deaths. She rouged her cheeks with fucus, a reddish-purplish paint. She darkened her lids, lashes, and brows with antimony or soot, and she emphasized milky skin by painting blue pigment over the veins on her chest and breasts.

As the Roman world gave way to the Christian one, women continued whitening their faces, dying their hair (blond was the preferred color), and rouging their cheeks

and lips with purple pigment. Three or four centuries after the death of Christ, they were still blackening their brows with soot and kohl. Jewish women in the ancient Middle East used cosmetics, including kohl moistened and drawn with a stick over tweezed, thinned brows.

THE MIDDLE AGES

In medieval times, upper-class women wanted to be as pale as lilies. To achieve a ghost-white appearance, they either had themselves bled or painted their faces with water-soluble paint. The women of sixth-century Spain painted their faces white. Spanish prostitutes indicated their profession by using pink paint. Eye makeup included shadows of various colorings— brown, taupe, gray. But the biggest change on a woman's face was her eyebrows . . . or lack of same.

In Europe, until the 1300s, the eyebrow was left in its natural state. An English poet in the thirteenth century described Milady's brows as "white between and not too near," and a French poet of the same period described the ideal woman as having brows

During the Middle Ages, women shaved both their eyebrows and their hairlines to give a pure, egglike look to their faces. By the early Renaissance, the old habits were dying, but eyebrows were still not allowed to flourish, and paintings of the period show an idealized but tiny brow. Madonna and Child with Saints John the Baptist and Catherine of Alexandria, ca. 1480–85, The Nerocchio de' Landi, Sienese, 1447–1500, The Norton Simon Foundation, Pasadena, California.

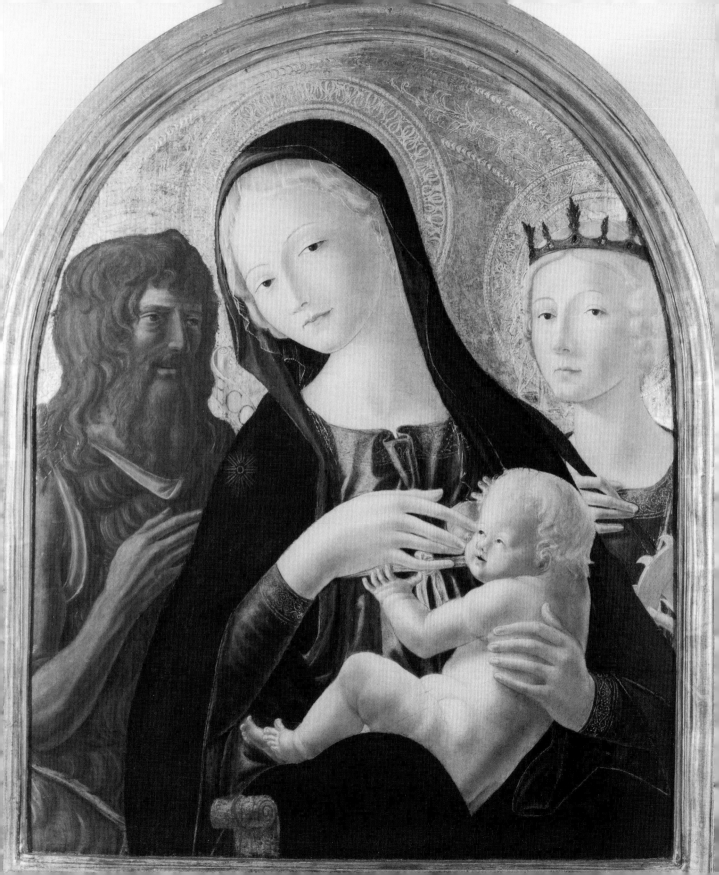

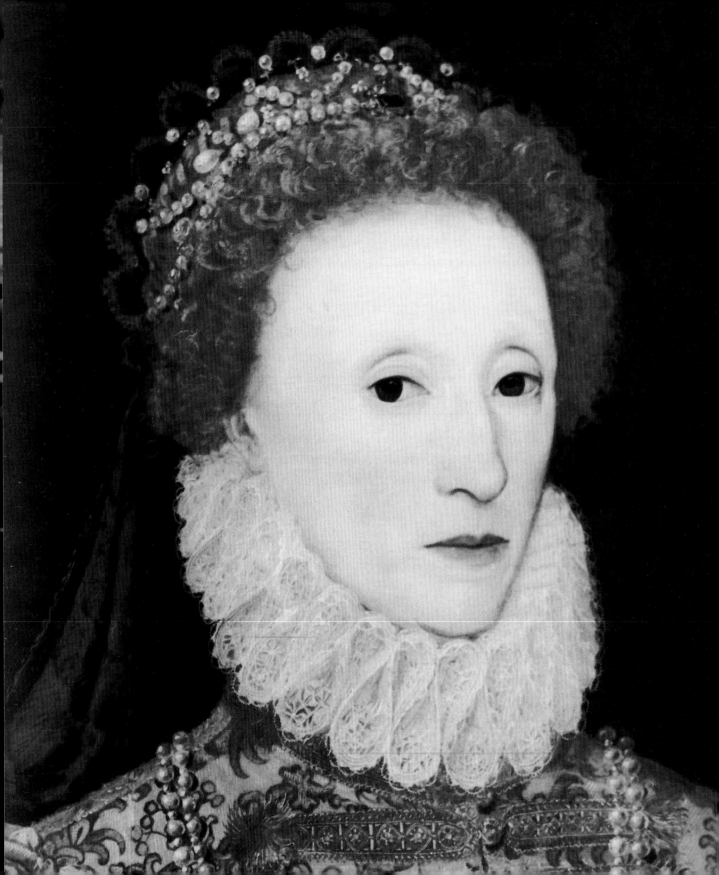

that were "brownish . . . narrow and delicate." But as the Middle Ages continued, the prevailing fashion was to tweeze the brow into a thin, narrow line. Pencil-thin brows crossed class lines. Chaucer wrote of the Carpenter's Wife in *The Canterbury Tales* as having "full small y-pulled were heres browes two/And they were bent. . . ."

A woman's crowning glory, her hair, was hidden under a headpiece. The effect, with the thin brow, was of a domelike forehead, much like the curvature of the perfect egg. Pale skin and a high, aristocratic forehead were admired. The look was demure, devoid of color or emphasis. Poor diet and lack of sunshine behind high castle walls contributed to this egglike countenance. Eventually, the hairline was shaved away and brows were eliminated altogether to allow for a high, broad forehead of pure white. To the modern eye, the resulting visage was insipid, helpless, devoid of all personality or sexual allure, but it made the medieval woman attractive to the knights who cherished the asexual pureness of courtly love. Only harlots painted up. It wasn't until the arrival of the mirror, crafted from highly polished silver or

Queen Elizabeth I painted her face with white ceruse and tweezed off most of her eyebrows, setting the fashion for the noblewomen of England. The effect was one of cold haughtiness, and her imperious spirit shows through in all the contemporary portraits of her. The "Darnley Portrait" of Elizabeth I (1533–1603) by an unknown artist, ca. 1575, Picture Library, National Portrait Gallery, London, England.

other metals, and the rise of the portrait painter toward the end of the Middle Ages, that there was a renewed interest in grooming and beauty. In the pastel-tinted portraits of Gothic medieval beauties in Northern Europe, a slight line of brow highlights a face surrounded by waves of delicate blond hair.

In other cultures during the Middle Ages, women painted heavily. In Byzantium, Theodora, the wife of the emperor Justinian, had traditional Eastern, kohl-rimmed eyes and a heavy, single eyebrow, accentuated with kohl. The mosaics in Ravenna, Italy, show her to have been stately, elegant, and striking with large eyes and an imperious look, aided and abetted by that unibrow.

In Asia at this time, the Japanese were developing traditional, ritualized makeups, later made famous by the Kabuki and Noh theaters. Fashionable Japanese women used white face paint, rouge, and red nail tints. They gilded their lower lips, blackened their teeth so they would not show, and shaved off their natural brows, painting new, perfect brows back on, usually over the site of the originals.

THE RENAISSANCE

By the time the Renaissance arrived, particularly in Italy, the Church was the patron saint of the arts, and the contemporary woman, painted as a saintly, chaste madonna in portraits, miniatures, and frescoes, was letting her natural eyebrows grow back. The fine art of the period documented the change.

In a fresco of a Florentine lady by Ghirlandaio, circa 1490, the lady's brows are still obliterated. As the century came to an end, brows made a bit of a comeback, but the fashionable woman was still tweezing them into a thin line. By the early 1500s, eyebrows returned to their natural fullness. In 1548, the Italian monk Firenzuola, writing in his *Dialogue on the Beauty of Women* (*Dialogo della bellezza delle donne*), described his ideal female:

> The forehead must be spacious. . . . The line of the brow should not be flat but curved in an arch toward the crown of the head, so gently that it scarce to be perceived; but from this boss of the temples, it should descend more straightly.

This very worldly monk also preferred that brows be of an ebony hue and the hairs be feathery and fine.

For most women of the time, painting brows for emphasis was almost nonexistent. Only prostitutes and the highborn used any cosmetics at all, preferring the traditional forms of eyebrow blackener: kohl, soot, or antimony.

In Elizabethan England, beauty customs were quite different. The High Renaissance woman wore restrictive, heavy, elaborate dresses, which were equipped with false hips and farthingales that held skirts out from tiny, corseted waists like a second set of arms. Clothing was ornate and decorated with sewn-on gems and pearls, and women wore ropes of pearls around their lily-white necks. The fashion of the day also dictated that the stiff, pleated ruff, adapted from Spanish fashion, frame the face. This put more emphasis on how the face was painted.

With her red hair and pale face, Queen Elizabeth I was an arresting fashion icon. Certainly, she was one of the first career women, giving up all thought of husband and children for her "job." When she was young, Elizabeth's ladies (who copied her look) lightened their skin, dyed their hair (often red, to match the queen's), exposed and lightened their breasts with white plaster, and tweezed or shaved their brows into nonexistence. They covered their faces with a paste of egg whites so they would look enameled, lined their eyes with kohl, and brightened them with a drop or two of the soporific belladonna.

As Elizabeth grew older, the paint on her face became like a mask. Her skin began to show the effects of faithful use of ceruse, the cosmetic made from toxic white lead. Toward the end of her life, her forehead became higher and higher while her hair became thinner and thinner. She resorted to wigs, shaved her eyebrows, and remained mostly in the dark of her chamber, refusing to attend to court duties or even look in the mirror.

Meanwhile, the Church was not thrilled with the beauty practices of the Elizabethan court. High Anglican prelates considered women who used false hair, false hips, makeup, and high-heeled shoes to be witches. But the court behaved as if the churchmen's recommendations of nondecorative piety didn't exist, and continued in its fashionable ways.

In other parts of Europe, women were using cosmetics again. Catherine de Medici spread the art of face painting from Italy to France. However, the cosmetics were toxic, not only destroying the skin, but sickening the wearer. Great numbers of women died from what were considered mysterious maladies. In an age of death by plague, childbirth, or smallpox, few people considered that cosmetics might have been the cause of some of these deaths.

The paints, for the most part, were poisonous, being made of mercury sulfide, powdered borax, ceruse, and Venetian turpentine. The fashionable woman considered ceruse essential to her beauty regimen—a fatal fad that persisted well into the eighteenth century. In the middle and late sixteenth century, women groomed their brows with tweezers and shaved their hairlines.

Toward the end of the sixteenth century, Italian women looked to Venice for their style direction. It was all about hair—gloriously golden, flowing hair. Venetian women painted themselves opulently and wore center-parted hair, earrings (a fairly new affectation), and a natural, unmolested brow. In the Golden Age of Venice, painters such as Titian and Tintoretto created gloriously shapely nudes with bleached blond hair and perfectly arched brows.

Portraits became more natural, less static and idealized, giving us a more accurate idea of what women really looked like.

THE RESTORATION

In England, after the death of Queen Elizabeth, during the Jacobean years, faces remained painted with white paste, and the lower lip became the focus of allure on the face. A protruding lower lip was considered the mark of a great beauty. Cheeks were rosy, and cream eye shadows in shades of blue or brown were worn, sometimes clear up to the eyebrow. Brows were darkened with soot or galena, but not tweezed.

Cosmetics and ostentation were set aside during the years after King Charles I was executed and Oliver Cromwell became Lord Protector of England in 1653. But the moment that royalist forces recovered the throne from the Protestant reformers and King Charles II was reinstated, painted women and men paraded in public, enjoying their new personal freedoms, not to mention debaucheries. Commented critic John Veely in 1654, "Women do begin to paint themselves, formerly an ignominious thing and used onlie by prostitutes."

The Restoration was a time of great flirtation between the sexes in the upper classes. Masks were tools of the game, and both men and women placed beauty patches, or "mouches," on their faces to trans-

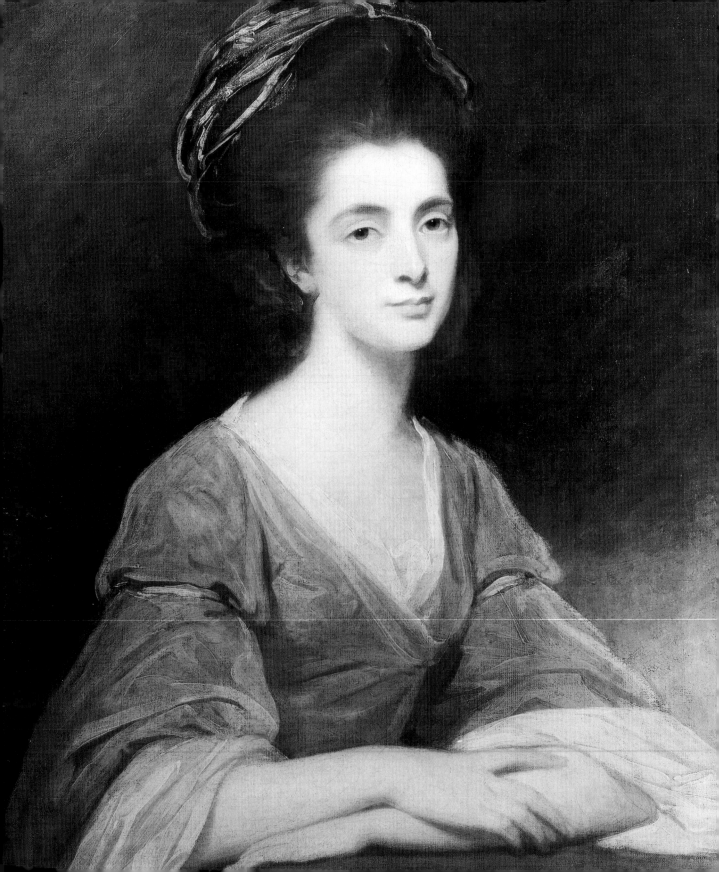

mit silent messages, depending upon where they were stuck. If the era was defined by any single cosmetic, it was the beauty patch, which could get very elaborate—butterflies and hearts and even miniature silhouettes of horse-drawn carriages made their way onto cheeks and foreheads and near the lips, eyes, and noses of the gentry. As for the eyebrows, they were left to grow as they pleased. The most prized women had wide, fleshy faces, full, red lips, protruding eyes, dark brows, dark hair, and double chins.

THE EIGHTEENTH CENTURY

In the French court circa 1700, women whitened their faces, emphasized the veins in their breasts with blue tracery (fine lines painted in watered-down blue ink), and penciled in their brows. In England at the turn of the century and through the Georgian period, the only women who did *not* paint, tweeze, and powder were the prostitutes. Cosmetics, which never really left Milady's toilette, were back with a vengeance, and so were eyebrows. They were tweezed and shaped and

By the mid-eighteenth century, most regal beauties of the British aristocracy no longer relied on false brows cut from mouse hide. Mrs. Charles Frederick (detail), ca. 1760, painted by Charles Romney, The Metropolitan Museum of Art, Fletcher Fund, 1945.

manipulated with brush and paint. As Tom Brown wrote in 1703 in *A Letter from the Dead to the Living*, "she shapes her eyebrows to a miracle." In *The Queen's Closet* in 1713, there were recipes for sweetening the breath, lightening freckles, and making a depilatory using the smashed shells of fifty-two eggs mixed with distilled water and used as a paste . . . presumably for facial hair and eyebrow reduction.

Regardless of what the fashionable women were doing in the privacy of their boudoirs, they were still the objects of satire, mostly because of their habit of covering their own eyebrows with fake ones cut from mouse hide. The portraits of the period show women with round, pink faces, double chins, and brows so arranged as to make them look perpetually surprised and quizzical.

Joseph Addison and Richard Steele didn't spare their critical vitriol in *The Spectator*. They decried women who painted as not being who they seemed, referring to the "Part of the Sex Who Paint" as "so exquisitely skillful this way that give them but a tolerable pair of eyes to set up with and they will make Bosom, Lips, Cheeks and Eye-brows by their industry." It was a bitter and incisive plaint, much like a twentieth-century husband who comments when his wife removes her hairpieces, false eyelashes, contact lenses, and padded bra: "Honey, I have to look for you in the drawer."

In one of his many commentaries, Jonathan Swift wrote of "Her eyebrows from a mouse's hide/Stuck on with art on either side." Matthew Prior composed no less than three verses about them. In "A Reasonable Affliction," he chortled, ". . . that the slattern had left in the Hurry and Haste/Her Lady's Complection and Eye-Brows at Calais." And he went into even greater detail and gales of laughter in a poem called "Another":

> Her Eye-brow box one morning lost
> (The best of Folks are oftenest crost)
> Sad Helen thus to Jenny said,
> Put me to bed then, Wretched Jane;
> Alas! When shall I rise again?
> I can behold no mortal owl
> For what's an eye without a brow . . .

By midcentury, the real beauties of the day were allowing their brows to grow back. While they still rouged and certainly patched, they also groomed their grown-back brows and arched them with judicious tweezing. Sir Harry Beaumont wrote of the ideal brow in 1752 in *Crito: A Dialogue on Beauty*, "The Eyebrows, well divided, rather full than thin, semicircular and broader in the middle than at the ends; of a neat turn, but not formal." To complete the picture, a woman should be blessed with a small rosebud of a mouth and plump cheeks.

Advice books with beauty recipes (written in the main by men, by the way) were sold in London toward the end of the century. A technique for blackening the brows appeared in a broadside that suggested rubbing the brows with ripe elderberries, burned cork (lampblack), burned ivory, or the black of frankincense. Those methods probably had their origin in the English translation of a commentary by a Frenchman named Antoine Le Camus, writing in *The Art of Preserving Beauty*. He suggested that brows be washed in a "decoction of Gall nuts wet with pencil or a brush dipped in a solution of green vitriol in which gum Arabic has been dissolved. They will dry black."

Gall nuts were an important ingredient in a number of recipes for hair and brow dye. The gall was a small oak tree that bore both acorns and small nodules of rounded woody substances known as galls, caused by the gall wasp laying eggs inside the bark of the tree. Galls were powdered or made into tincture and ointments. They were a powerful astringent, used medically for swelling, inflammation, and dysentery . . . and obviously, for tinting hair.

Fashions of the century were influenced not only by the great beauties and the portrait painters, but by world travelers who came back bearing tales of the so-called exotic civilizations. Letter writers reported from Greece, Russia, and as far away as

Following the Kabuki theatrical tradition, Japanese courtesans obliterated their natural eyebrows with white face paint and replaced them with perfect renderings of eyebrows that were a combination of blackener brushed on over red paint. Courtesan Holding Fan *(detail), ca. 1793, Kitagawa Utamaro (1753–1806), The Metropolitan Museum of Art, Rogers Fund, 1922.*

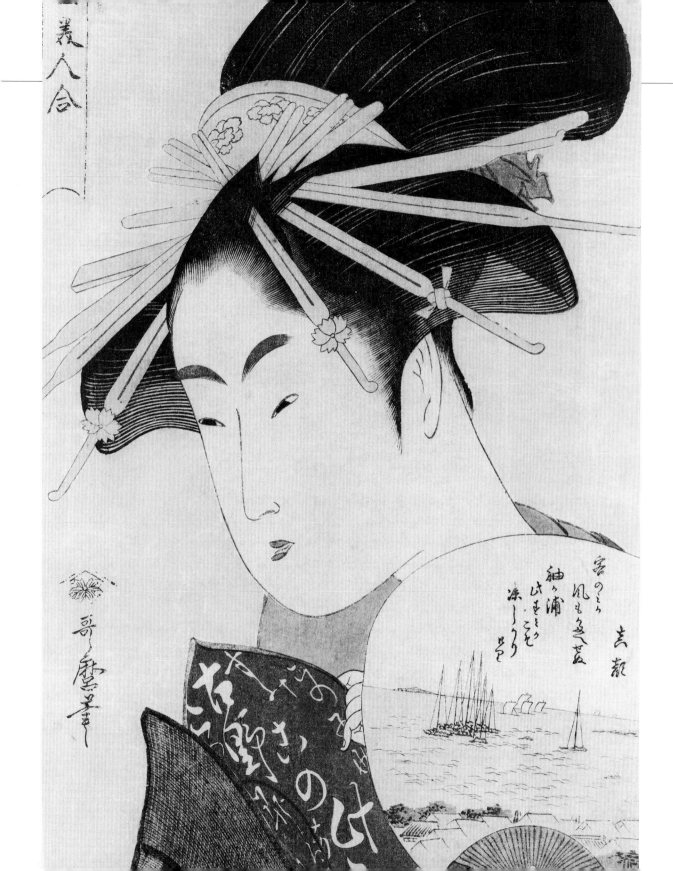

Japan. In Greece, one correspondent wrote, women used soot inside their lashlines and on their brows. Catherine the Great of Russia, it was said, had a full face, a double chin, and full, quite natural brows. Turkish women were said to dye their brows with a black tincture. The women of the Orient, particularly the Chinese, were admired for their small eyes. Girls plucked their brows continually, to keep them narrow and wide apart. In Japan the traditions of the Kabuki and Noh theaters dictated a ritualized face that was neutralized with an allover wash of white paint. In order to be seen in a darkened theater, eyebrows were blocked out with white and new ones were painted on above the natural brow.

In France, as the century wore on, the great beauties, including Madame Pompadour and Madame Du Barry, indulged in heavy makeup. In the cosseted world of Louis XIV, high foreheads were an emblem of beauty, and if a woman didn't come by hers naturally, she removed the offending low hairline with tweezers. To prevent their children from growing unattractively low hairlines, mothers washed their brows with walnut oil.

Meanwhile, back in Britain, "macaronis," fashionable young blades who had traveled to Italy, affected Italian dress. Considered foppish in the extreme, these young men painted like women—wearing patches, powder, elaborate wigs, and artificially darkened brows.

In the waning years of the century, fashion in both England and France was all about hair and hats—great mounds of hair piled under elaborately plumed and flowered hats with huge brims, tied with yards of ribbon under the chin. In the 1780s, while some women in England continued to wear false brows made of mouse hide, Marie Antoinette retired to her estate, Le Petit Trianon, where she kept sheep and chickens, took off her panniers and gems, washed the powder out of her hair, and tried to live a simple, bucolic life. Her search for the pastoral pleasures ushered in a fashion for the natural, unadorned face, although at the more formal Versailles, the court women still painted and wore coiffures that defied gravity. Their hair was done up in such fantastical display, powdered and greased with bear fat or pomade, that they would not take these hairy confections apart for days. Often they were besieged by bugs, weevils, and lice, and owned long, pointed instruments like knitting needles designed to scratch the scalp without disturbing the coiffure. There was a high price to pay for fashion in the final days of Louis XIV's reign.

The French valued the long, swanlike neck (the perfect target, by the way, as Madame La Guillotine took the heads of the aristocracy with the fall of the monarchy in 1793), rouged cheeks, and the stylized coiffure. Eyebrows were almost an afterthought, perhaps a harbinger of what was to come as the new century dawned: a period of naturalness.

THE EARLY NINETEENTH CENTURY

In the early 1800s, the beauty pendulum had swung nearly 180 degrees from the ultimate artifice of powdered hair, false brows, rouged cheeks, and beauty patches to a more ethereal look. Women still painted, but with a lighter hand, in keeping with their sheer, gossamer gowns, no foundation garments, bare legs, and short, cropped, curly hair.

During the French Revolution, many aristocrats escaped to England. This would have a huge effect on English beauty. The same could be said of the reign of Napoleon. Despite the fact that the British were at war with him for nearly twenty-five years, Englishwomen could not get enough of French fashion and cosmetic artistry. If Marie Antoinette had set the pace for the French court of Louis XIV, it was Josephine Beauharnais, the daughter of Caribbean planters, who captivated the future emperor of France and established the signature look of the Empire. She used rouge to combat her lack of natural glow and cut her hair short to frame and emphasize her expressive, wide-set eyes.

While one fashionable Englishwoman wrote that women "should be content to leave her eyes as she found them," decrying penciling or staining brows as "clumsy tricks of attempted deception" that elicited "contempt for bad taste," most British women faithfully followed the fashion of the French Empire. Those considered most beautiful, like Lady Emma Hamilton, mistress of Lord Nelson, commander of the British fleet, had small, rounded faces, rosebud mouths, and upturned, retroussé noses. Faces were still whitened with cosmetics made of white lead, and hair was powdered and curled like that of a French poodle. Eyes were left bare of makeup, and brows were untweezed and natural.

THE VICTORIAN ERA

You would think that in the era of the plain Jane, cosmetics and overgrooming would be an unpleasant reminder of another age. Perhaps the early Victorians, with their severe center-parted hair, covered ears, poke bonnets, and heavy, ungroomed brows, seemed like a joyless lot. They dressed and undressed in the dark, spent long hours indoors, and when they did go abroad in the daytime, hid their complexions from exposure to sun and air under parasols and bonnets with face-obscuring brims. But despite their pale, neurasthenic faces, they fluffed pearl powder on their noses and used scents made of elderflower and rosewater. Perhaps surreptitiously, they groomed their brows with lampblack mixed with ointment and applied with a fine camel's hair brush, known as a pencil, which lead to the term "penciling in the brow." Men were known to use "pencils" on their brows, too.

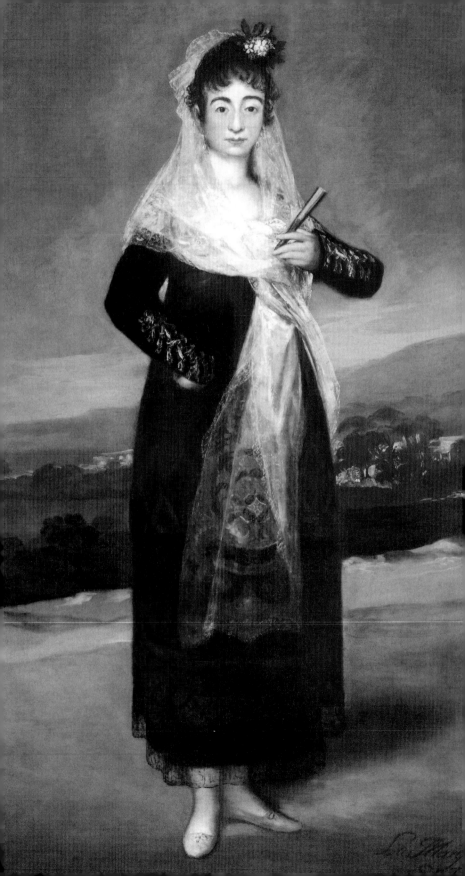

The Victorians were a society that traveled. Again, in letters and diaries, they observed the mores and the fashions in lands whose customs were quite foreign to their own. Reported a Lady Sheil in *Glimpses of Life in Persia*, "All Kajars have naturally large, arched eyebrows, but not satisfied with this, the women enlarge them by doubling their *real* size with great streaks of antimony." Travelers also reported that the Jewish women of Turkey, circa 1833, blackened their brows and even wore artificial ones made of animal hair (probably in keeping with the Orthodox Jewish tradition of masking one's natural hair under a wig, or *sheidel*). Recipes for making eye-darkening kohl came from Arabia. One instructed: Fill a lemon rind with plumbago (leadwort) and burned copper and place it in the fire until it turns to carbon; pound it in a mortar with coral, sandalwood, ambergris, batwings, and a chameleon cooked to a cinder; and wet it with rosewater.

In Japan during the nineteenth century, the rise of the geisha brought even more stylization to make-ups, which were traditionally ritualized by the Kabuki and Noh theaters. The geisha first applied

During and after the Napoleonic Wars of the early nineteenth century, the Spanish noblewoman used arsenic-based white ceruse makeup on her face with a dash of cheek color, but her eyes and eyebrows were left in their natural state. The J. Paul Getty Museum, Los Angeles, Francisco José de Goya y Lucientes, Portrait of the Marquesa de Santiago *(detail), 1804, oil on canvas, 82 ½ by 49 ¾ inches.*

pink makeup on her face to neutralize her features. Then she brushed white chalk gently over it. All was blended together for a finish like porcelain. Rouge was applied by brush with a very light hand on the cheeks, eyelids, and by the side of the nose. The white color was brushed carefully from eyebrows and lashes. Finally, the brows were painted first with red and then overpainted in black, and rubbed a bit until some of the red showed through. The finished face was quite doll-like and sweet, not to mention accommodating and helpless.

By the 1840s in Britain and America, women could find recipes for home-brewed cosmetics in publications like *Godey's Lady's Book*. Brows, for instance, could be dyed with a mixture of sulfate of iron, distilled water, gum water, and eau de cologne, deemed by the fashionable book as too irritating to use on the lashes.

Other beauty "experts" included the fabulous Lola Montez, a self-styled interpreter of Spanish dance. Montez was born in Ireland and became, after a very speckled career in which she was booed off the stage in London, the mistress of both Franz Liszt and King Louis I of Bavaria. A beautiful and influential woman who died at forty-three of paralysis (brought on, wags of the time liked to whisper, by overindulgence in poisonous cosmetics), she made quite a name for herself as the power behind the throne of Bavaria.

Of course, a great beauty like Lola had to share her secrets. She wrote a beauty book advising that eye makeup was "absurd and ruinous to beauty" and "an

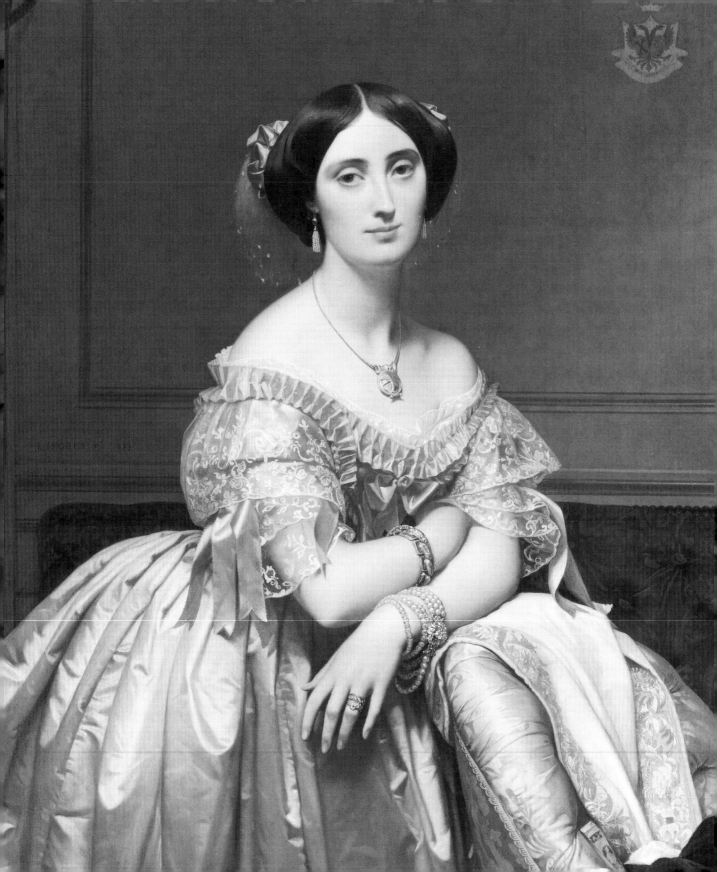

THE EYEBROW THROUGH HISTORY

insult to nature." She advocated darkening the brows only if "a woman had the misfortune of diseases or otherwise, to have deficient eye-brows. She may delicately supply the want as far as she can, with artificial penciling." She warns, however, that the penciling should be as close to nature as possible.

Midcentury in England, as the Pre-Raphaelite brotherhood of artists led by the poet Dante Gabriel Rossetti was coming into fashion, the plain woman, totally unadorned, was looked upon as desirable. In *The Art of Beauty,* Mrs. H. R. Haweis described the ideal Pre-Raphaelite fashionable (or was she an anti-fashionable?) with her "pallid face with protruding upper lip. Green eyes, a squint, square eyebrows . . . now is the time for plain women." This cynosure of homeliness had a demure, ghostly white face with long, center-parted hair that was allowed to fall free. The Pre-Raphaelite woman affected melancholy eyes under beetled, heavy brows that gave the appearance

Throughout Europe, Queen Victoria's prim, buttoned-up influence was so pervasive that women used very few cosmetics on their faces and allowed themselves only a dash of scent. Victorian-era women used loops of their center-parted hair to cover their ears and let their eyebrows return to their natural state. Ladies of the period were urged to be retiring, demure, and quite dependent on their husbands and fathers. Josephine-Eleonore-Marie-Paulina de Galard de Brassac de Bearn, Princesse de Broglie (1825–1867) *(detail), ca. 1853, Jean-Auguste-Dominique Ingres (1780–1867), The Metropolitan Museum of Art, Robert Lehman Collection, 1975.*

of a great (and romantic) sadness, mystery, and drama. Or . . . great suffering.

But suffering for beauty had been a long-standing custom through the ages. And by 1874, with her waist corseted into the width of two hands, the mid-Victorian woman had decided that a little bit of grooming and care wasn't going to hurt her. In 1875, another self-styled beauty expert, Dr. Pierre Cazenove, wrote in *Female Beauty: Of the Art of Human Decoratio*n, that eyebrows "to be handsome, should be well-furnished with hair, moderately thick, curved and form a line in the shape of an arch. The head [of the brow] should have more hair and numerous short hairs should lie in and out. The two eyebrows should never meet, and though one sees them perfectly united, it is at present day looked upon as a deformity." Cazenove also advocated grooming brows with a soft toothbrush dipped in cologne-scented water.

But as much as the good doctor decried artificially blackening the brow, he did supply a pair of recipes for brow dye: for black brows, gall nuts and oil mixed with ammoniac salt, in vinegar, applied at night and rinsed off in the morning. For brown brows: lead filings dissolved in vinegar, boiled together, shaken and cooled, stroked on at night, and washed off in the morning.

The Victorian woman's eyebrow required little artifice at all. Obviously tweezed or very thin brows were not in style. Eyebrows, like hair, were considered lovely if they were very thick and very dark. In

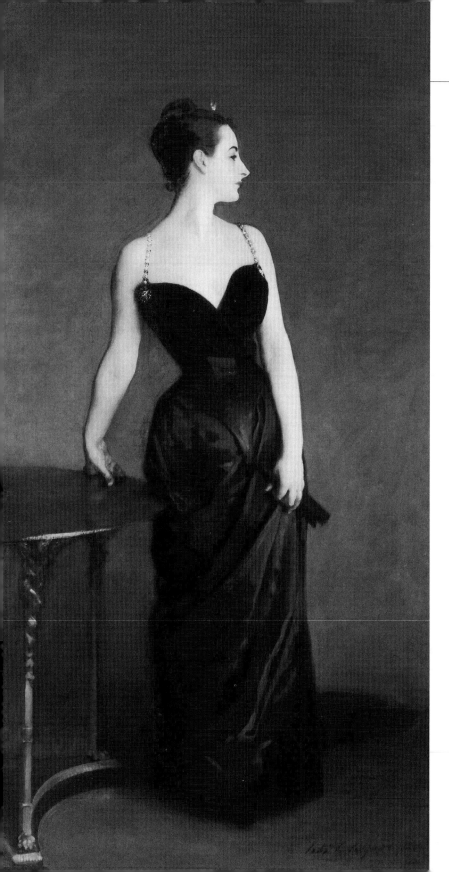

an attempt to thicken a brow, a contemporary beauty expert named Margaret Cunliffe recommended rubbing them with an infusion of white wine and mint leaves. Haweis's *The Art of Beauty*, meanwhile, advocated small brushes for grooming brows and keeping them "well-arched to give the face an air of serenity." Also recommended: brushing brows with oil before retiring for the night. The period was thick with beauty advice books and women whose profession was to minister to the fairer sex. To darken brows, women were advised to hold a small piece of wood in a candle flame, rub the excess carbon off, and use the residue on their brows. One writer said: "Bear in mind that this is a very delicate operation and should be done with a steady hand, as nothing looks more horrible than to see the large black band very badly outlined, which passes with some women for eyebrows."

John Singer Sargent captured the beauty of La Belle Époque in his portrait of Madame X, whose imperious carriage was heightened by her carefully manicured brows. Madame X (Madame Pierre Gautreau), *ca. 1882–1884, John Singer Sargent (1856–1925), The Metropolitan Museum of Art, Arthur H. Hearn Fund, 1916.*

Women's ideas of cosmetics had grown quite conservative at this time, but dyeing and tinting were thought to be more acceptable and ladylike than the use of temporary, wash-off cosmetics. Eyebrow pencils in black, dark brown, and blond that came directly from the stage were deemed far too obvious. But careful tweezing was recommended if brows met over the nose, which was thought to make women look angry, not sweet, coy, and diffident.

Late Victorian women also emphasized their brows with India ink or with frankincense black, which was made by dipping frankincense, pitch, resin, and gum mastic onto hot coals, collecting the colored smoke in a large paper funnel, scraping off the black powder residue, mixing it with fresh elderberry juice or eau de cologne, and applying it with a camel's hair brush. A woman could also hold a fine China saucer over a candle flame to collect the carbon and apply it to her brows and lashes with a matchstick. The very proper Victorian could then get rid of the evidence by burning the paper funnel or simply washing the dish. Whew. At-home beauty was very labor intensive.

Toward the end of the 1800s, things began changing rapidly. Morals and customs were shedding their tightly corseted, forbidding ways. The male-dictated prison that femininity had been locked in for the better part of the century was losing its hold on the contemporary woman as the availability of commercially made, mass-marketed beauty aids made it easier to adorn one's face, not to mention that their use was more socially acceptable in the first place. Chemist shops and Sears Roebuck shops stocked face powder, skin-care creams, and eyebrow pencils. In the 1890s, the Sears Roebuck catalog advertised Almond Nut Cream, Secret of Ninon (a bleaching concoction for freckle removal), powder puffs, and depilatories. *Vogue* magazine had started offering beauty advice to its readers. Late in the nineteenth century, future beauty queen Helena Rubinstein emigrated from Poland to Australia and, soon after the turn of the twentieth century, set up shop in London.

As the new century approached, with its fabled Edwardian beauties, Belle Époque ornamentation, premonitions of the coming Great War, and silent picture industry, women were about to break out of their Victorian corsets with a vengeance. The Edwardians, at any rate, knew a little something about feminine allure and celebrated it full force, with powdered faces and eyebrows groomed and arched with an elegance not seen in the annals of fashion. It was a brand-new century, and a whole new era of beauty for the emerging emancipated woman.

THE
TWENTIETH
CENTURY

ONE HUNDRED YEARS OF EYEBROW TRANSFORMATION

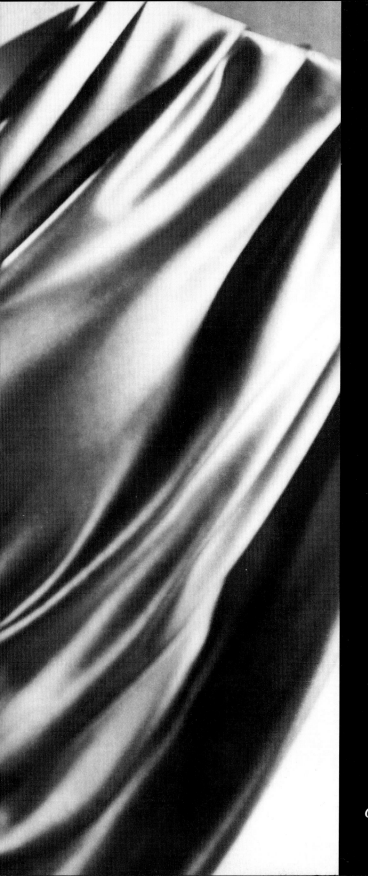

The story of the eyebrow's progress through the twentieth century parallels the story of women's independence. In the 1920s, when women started paying attention to their faces and their freedom, brows were tweezed, narrowed, and groomed with great élan and creativity. In the 1930s, in the midst of a worldwide depression, when fairy-tale images of the Ideal, the Perfect, the Elevated were sought after to alleviate the penury of no jobs and few prospects, eyebrows were tweezed nearly into nothingness and redrawn. In the 1940s, during World War II, when women not only kept the home fires burning, they stoked the defense machine, America's wholesome Rosie the Riveters were too busy to maintain narrow, labor-intensive eyebrows, so they let them grow out. And in the postwar years, when Christian Dior's soignée New Look put women back in girdles and corsets, the eyebrow experienced its most stylish and high-maintenance decade yet. Like the Roaring Twenties, the Swingin' Sixties was another profligately free decade when creativity spawned a painted eye and a brow decorated with lace, feathers, glitter, and even diamonds. In the 1970s, the Disco Decade of Dreadful Taste, women were at their tweezers again, manicuring their brows into cramped little tadpoles or flighty commas. The Go-Go Eighties were years of more is more, and the brow took its cue from big hair and big shoulders as career women attacked boardroom doors in their power suits. And in the 1990s, the eyebrow was once again a malleable fashion accessory, designed now by superstar makeup artists who determined The Look of fashion model, trophy wife, and screen star . . . and, eventually, the rest of us.

Carole Lombard

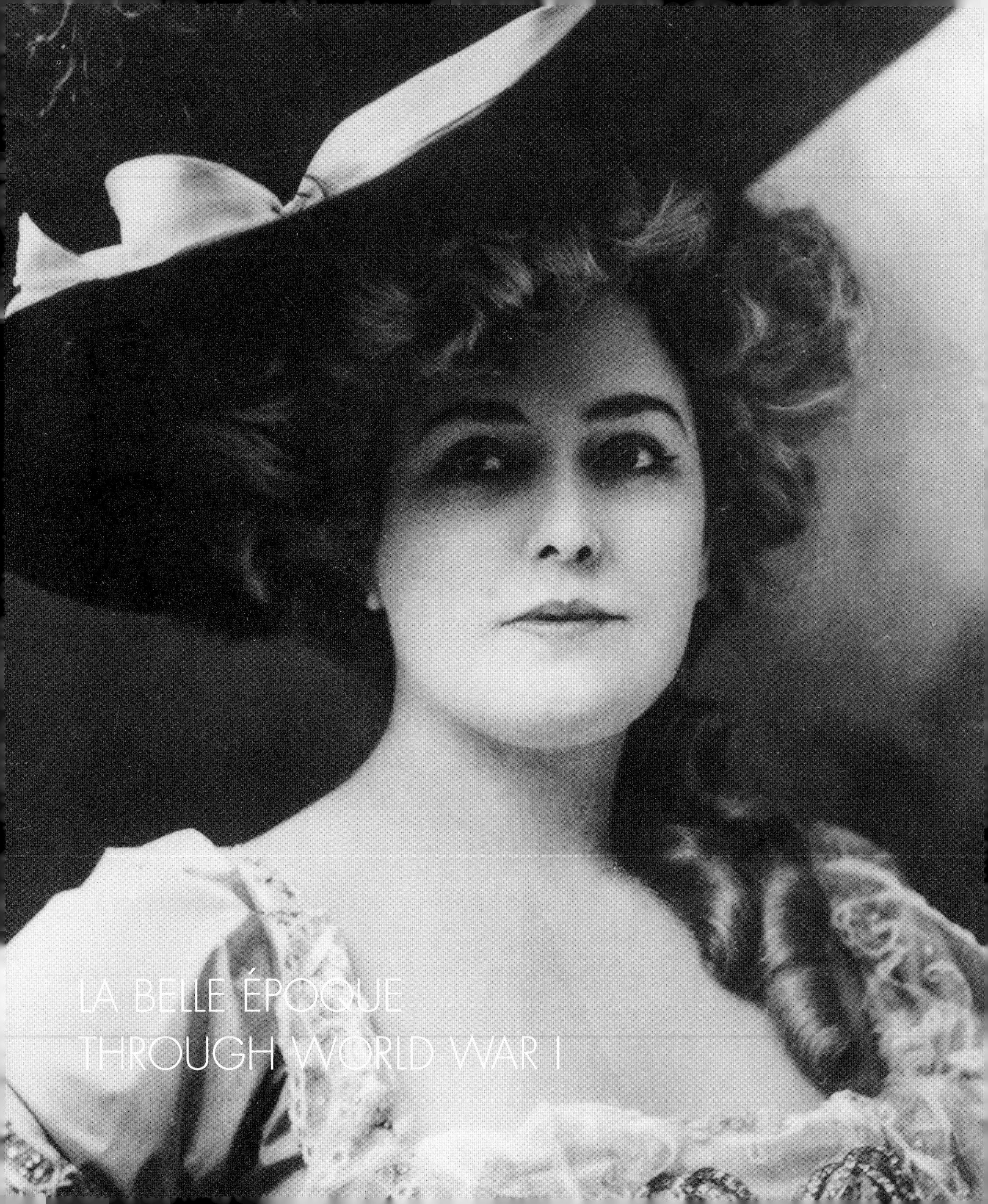

LA BELLE ÉPOQUE THROUGH WORLD WAR I

At the turn of the century, the eyebrow was a wild thing—a forest of hairs that marched across milady's nose or bristled angrily from her face. Only the very decadent, expensive courtesan or highborn society dame even dared groom her brow.

Yet, the future was at hand and social observers such as the English wit Max Beerbohm could write wry commentaries about what was becoming obvious. In 1896, Beerbohm penned an article, "In Defense of Cosmetics," in which he said, with tongue planted firmly in cheek:

> For behold! The Victorian era comes to an end. . . . No longer is a lady of fashion blamed if, to escape the outrageous persecution of the time, she fly for sanctuary to the toilet table, and if a damsel, plying her mirror, be sure that with brush and pigment she can trick herself into more charm, we are not angry. . . .

Queen Victoria died in 1901 and by then, the elegant excesses of La Belle Époque were in full force. The Edwardians, those patrician, stylish, highly mobile folks who sailed back and forth to Europe as if the Atlantic were their own private fishpond, were pleasure-loving, high-consuming style-setters. It was

Lillian Russell was a music hall performer, socialite, and mistress of New York bon vivant Diamond Jim Brady. Like the women of her time, she used cosmetics and scent and groomed her eyebrows with tweezers and black pencil.

the era of bounteous, overdone, buxom women of questionable repute such as Lillian Russell, who displayed groomed and tweezed brows along with her angelic face, soufflé mounds of blond hair, and voluptuous figure, and the Jersey Lily, Lillie Langtry, mistress to King Edward VII, whose style and makeup were copied by the masses.

At the World's Fair in Paris in 1900, the *haut monde* met the *beau monde* when artists like Klimt and Munch idealized women as uncorseted, bohemian wood nymphs with their hair unburdened and their eyebrows, furry and untouched. It was also a time when intrepid American heiresses (so eloquently limned in Edith Wharton's *The Buccaneers*) were sent to Britain and the Continent to snag a title for their robber baron fathers.

The reigning, wellborn, and proper beauties of the day were Queen Alexandra, wife of Edward VII of England, and Consuelo Vanderbilt, the American heiress who became the Duchess of Marlborough. As painted by John Singer Sargent, the duchess was a haughty beauty with a wasp waist, full bosom, and a strong, exquisite face—a true oval—with a heart-shaped mouth, huge eyes, and strikingly thick and well-arched eyebrows. From Sargent's portrait and contemporary photographs, it is obvious that the duchess took very good care of herself, wore cosmetics, and groomed her naturally thick brows. As for Queen Alexandra, she was a dedicated follower of fashion who shocked her subjects by wearing cosmetics—cheek color, eyebrow pencil, lash blackener, and powder—but only for evening fêtes.

Certainly women were getting restless as the new century progressed. They were still idealized by artists like Charles Dana Gibson, whose Gibson Girl was the picture of industry and respectability in her high-necked, frilly white shirtwaist, unbustled skirt, and glossy topknot of long, thick hair. Young women were entering the workforce as clerks in the new department stores or as stenographers in high-rise offices. They took trams by themselves or rode bicycles (with their split skirts designed by Amelia Bloomer) and then used their incomes to buy cosmetics, such as Fard Italien, an eyebrow pencil.

Before 1900, there were few commercial cosmetics available to the women who wanted to use them. And a majority of those that were sold in catalogs and in a growing number of private beauty salons were of questionable purity. Women were still cooking up cosmetics in their kitchen sinks and passing recipes for cheek color, lip pomade, skin whiteners, and eyebrow darkeners from mother to daughter. Bismuth was recommended to lighten skin; walnut leaves for eye-brightening salves. Burned matchsticks still blackened brows and lashes, but the early Edwardian woman could purchase cold cream, Vaseline, and Yardley's Lavender Water at her local dry goods store.

Suddenly, a spate of products appeared on the market in addition to cold cream: Rouge de Théâtre to redden cheeks, Japanese rice powder, Blanc de Perles to lighten skin tone, birch balsam to cover pockmarks caused by smallpox, and pencils for lids and brows. Women's magazines endorsed them gladly and benefited from the resulting advertising revenues. In 1900, American *Vogue* became the first and last word for beauty advice. *Vogue* heartily recommended eye makeup, including cosmetic crayons to deepen the shade of the lashes. They came in five shades—black, brown, chestnut, blond, and navy blue—with a cake of wax that had to be warmed over an oil lamp before using.

Eyebrows in the early 1900s were slightly groomed—that is, women were darkening them with pencil and shaping them to echo the contour of the eye. A contemporary beauty expert interpreted the shape of the brow and assigned to it personality traits. For instance, she said, if a woman's brows were too straight, her face took on an astonished air; if her brows met at the nose in a hard, fixed expression, she had a jealous nature.

Whether commercial cosmetics were readily available or not, the beauty experts were all of an accord. Cosmetics *should* be seen . . . but barely. Writing in *Le Bréviaire de la Femme*, Parisian Comptesse de Tramer declared that makeup should be "invisible." "Cream [the face]," she ordered, "then wipe the face, then take a powder made of white pearl, then apply rouge with a rabbit's foot. Make a paste of cloves to put on the eyelids and eyebrows, wiping it off with a finger." Lashes, she suggested, could be lengthened with a secret "from the harem": China ink diluted with rosewater.

Internationally, culture and custom changed from country to country. In England makeup was the province of the highborn or the prostitute. And only the latter would wear powder, rouge, lip color, and eyebrow pencil *before* sundown. Across the Channel in Paris, attitudes toward racy *femmes* were quite different. It was the French courtesan, also often an actress or a music hall performer, who set the styles of the day. Women such as Liane de Pougy, Émilienne d'Alençon, and La Belle Otéro had their social lives and personal styles celebrated in *Le Figaro* and *La Revue*. Their heavy makeups came directly from the stage; they adapted theatrical techniques and products to their faces, using lampblack or Fard Italien for their manicured eyebrows.

If the future of the eyebrow seemed to be dim and undefined before 1910, it was not for a woman's lack of exposure to what the fashionable and the con-

Oscar Wilde compared actress and reigning beauty Lillie Langtry with Helen of Troy. She had pale violet eyes, an exquisite complection, and dark eyebrows that she groomed lightly.

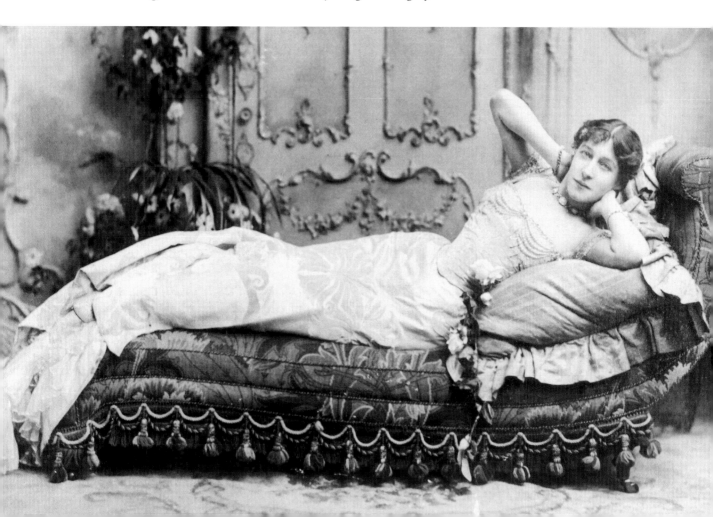

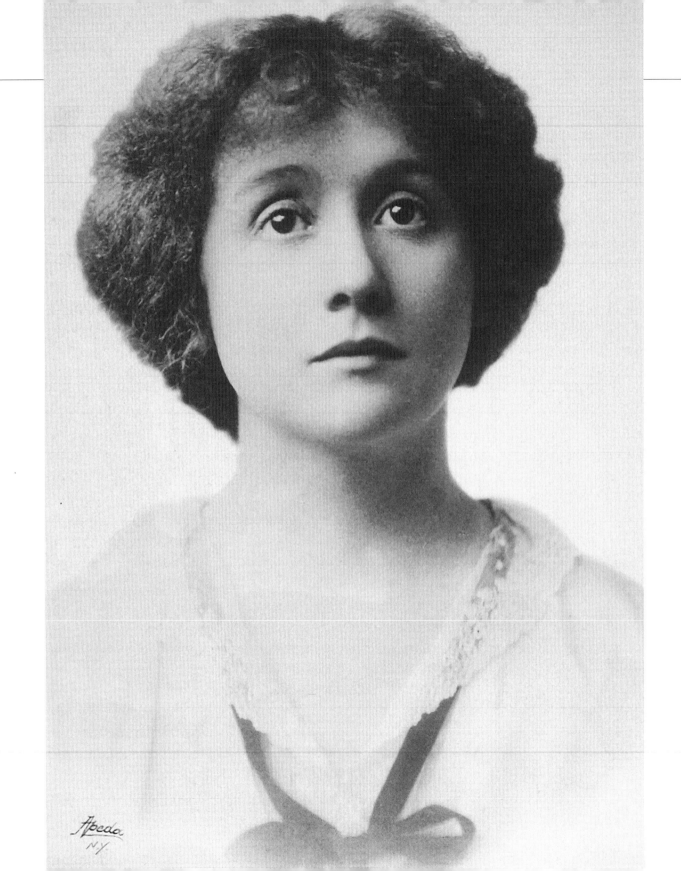

troversial were wearing both on their bodies and on their faces. The fashion magazine was gaining in importance. Primarily, however, it was from the stage—theater and vaudeville—that the next wave of beauty was coming.

Stage cosmetics circa 1900 were still crude affairs. Illumination in theaters came from dimly flickering gaslights. To be seen across the footlights, an actor had to exaggerate his makeup. Black pencils in tubes—Crayons d'Italie or Fard Italien—lined eyes and darkened brows and lashes. Chalk and red carmine pigment colored the face. The invention of incandescent lighting necessitated improved products and a lighter hand. Greasepaint by Hubert of Berlin was used and in America, Max Factor, who by this time had emigrated and settled in Los Angeles, sold stage makeup out of a small store on Central Avenue, including greasepaint, rouge, eyebrow pencils, and eyeliners.

When theatrical makeup changed—when it was refined, that is—the influence of stage and ballet maquillage translated commercially. Before 1910, the cinema was still considered a novelty. The age of the silent film goddess was nearly ten years away.

In 1909, a unique theatrical event was to transform all standards of beauty. The Ballets Russes, under the direction of the flamboyant Serge

The first directors did not pay attention to the emotional possibilities of the eyebrow. The eyes and brows of silent film actress Bessie Barriscale are totally natural.

Diaghilev, arrived in Paris with the electrifying Nijinsky and the delicate Anna Pavlova dancing in such daring productions as *Salomé*, *L'Après-midi d'un faune*, and *Narcisse*. The company's influence instigated daring trends in both fashion and beauty and had a massive effect on Western fashion. Couturiers like Paul Poirot adapted the looks designed for the stage by Léon Bakst and Romain de Titroff, aka Erté. Poirot's clothes were particularly dazzling. They were relaxed silhouettes in rich Eastern colors—reds, golds, ochers, violets—created from sumptuous fabrics.

To match the drama of the new styles, women changed their makeups. Where fashionable women had once adapted the ladylike cosmetic colors of the musical comedy and vaudeville stage, the polite powder-blue eye shadow and baby-pink mouth, maquillage was radicalized by the Ballets Russes' groundbreaking production design. Fashion-hungry women from Paris to New York to Hollywood copied the look: the darkly maquillaged eye with its Asian cast and the fantastic, graphic eyebrow. Eyes were encircled with heavy black liner; the slanted doe eye of the ballerina was copied. Lines penciled both under and over the eye met in the outward corners in elongated triangles. The exaggerated almond shape was mirrored by the upward and outward sweep of brows that resembled the exotic Mandarin, the sloe-eyed vamp, the harem houri. Using pencil kohl (called *kajal*), women added angry black slashes to their brows. The low, flat eyebrows that skimmed the top of the eye beetled the brow. What was supposed to look sexy and mysterious also turned a sweet visage into that of an angry virago.

In America, *Vogue* magazine acknowledged the trend by informing readers about beauty rituals from romanticized, faraway places. They were told of Turkish and Circassian women, who employed henna to pencil their eyes and brows, and of the Arabs of the desert, whose women blackened the edges of their eyelids and their brows with dark powder. The medicinal as well as the cosmetic virtues of *kajal* were described in detail. There were printed reports of the popularity in the Middle East of the unibrow, which was described as a sign of beauty in that part of the world.

Meanwhile, in the United States, Max Factor founded his cosmetics company, supplying makeup to vaudevillians and touring actors. Factor also introduced eye shadows and eyebrow pencils for the public, which he sold in his Central Avenue shop as the Max Factor Society line.

Existing greasepaints were adequate for the primitive technical demands of those days, but actors wanted a cosmetic that was not as masklike when it dried. And with the burgeoning film industry at Factor's backdoor in Hollywood, the medium called for even more radical changes in cosmetics.

What actors used onstage did not work for film. Stage makeups cracked under the hot lights that are necessary for making movies. Actors, painted pale and ghostly, looked as if they were wearing death masks. In 1914, Factor came to their rescue with the first of many cosmetic inventions that eventually hit the commercial market. He called his innovation "flexible greasepaint," a makeup that moved with the actor's face, allowing it to register true emotion on screen. The result: For such facially mobile players as Charlie Chaplin, Roscoe "Fatty" Arbuckle, and Buster Keaton, the new flexible greasepaint freed up expression and allowed the camera to dolly in closer to capture a full range of emotion.

With the development of the cinematic close-up, the eyes and eyebrows became the most important components of the face. The early screen sirens—Pola Negri, Theda Bara, and Gloria Swanson—benefited from their close-ups and spawned a generation of women who avidly copied their Femme Fatale look.

In 1914, Theda Bara, a nice Jewish girl from Cincinnati, Ohio (her studio-created name was an anagram for "Arab Death"), starred in *A Fool There Was*, as the first of the vamps (short for "vampire"). In makeup created by the newly arrived Polish émigré Helena Rubinstein, she was exotic and forbidding. Her complexion had a deathly white pallor; her brows were heavy and blackened. They fled straight across the tops of her eyes, which were pools of black, surrounded by heavy kohl. With eyebrows penciled on in a downward swoop toward her nose, Bara

Theda Bara was the first film vamp. Makeup artists applied heavy kohl and mascara to turn Bara's eyes into burning black coals, and her brows flew angrily across her eyes in definitive slashes. Rather than looking sexy, Bara just looked mad as the devil, which was probably the idea.

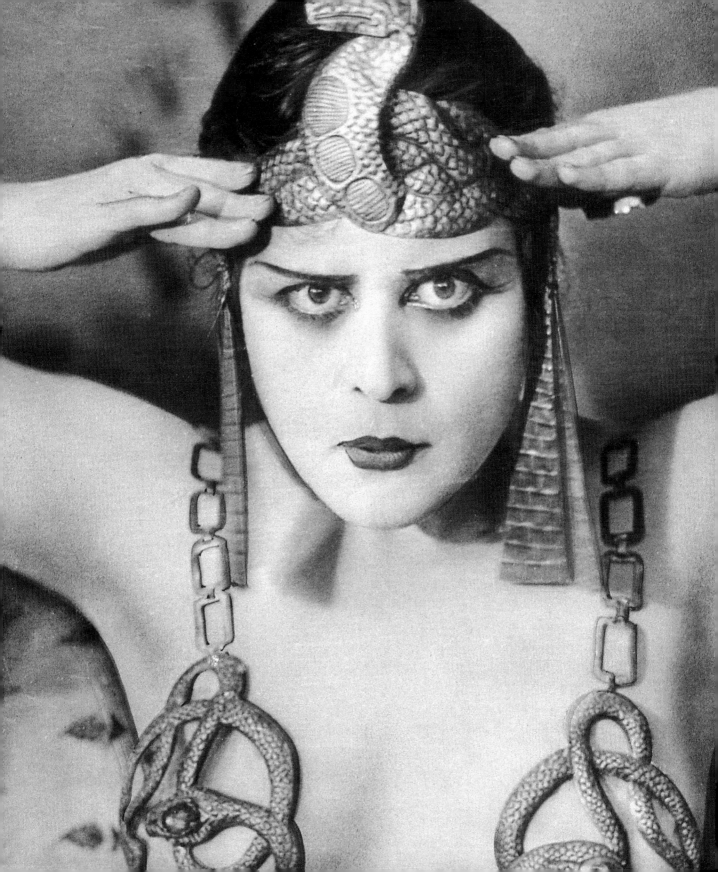

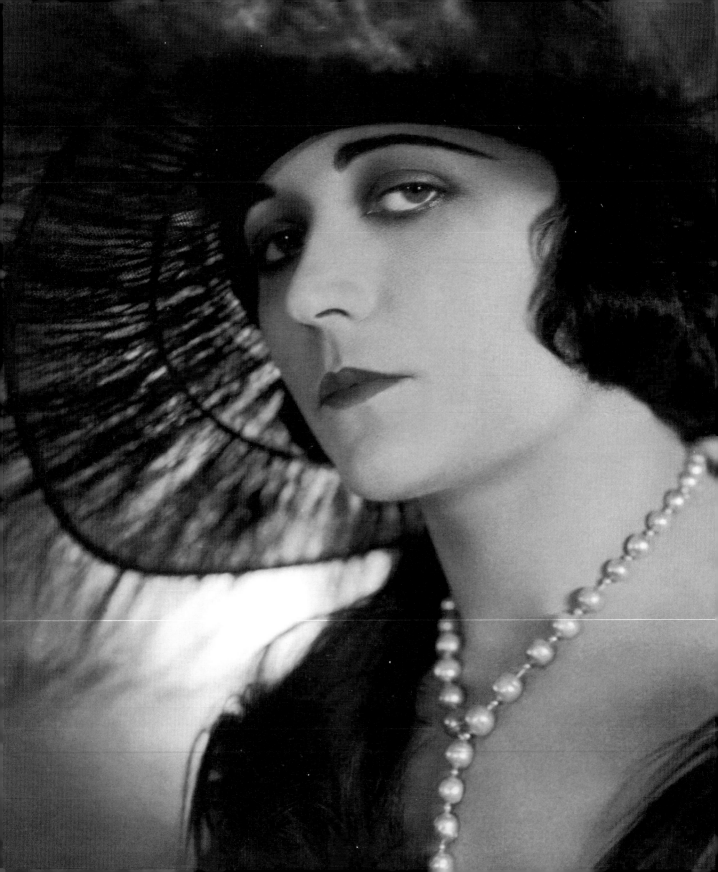

looked fearsome, angry, with the don't-mess-with-me attitude of the Femme Fatale that was both intriguing and repellent at the same time.

Pola Negri, a Polish-born actress who moved to Germany to work with Ernst Lubitsch, married both a count and a prince. By the time she started acting in pictures, she had learned to use her eyes as part of her exotic persona. They were dark and deep-set, kohled with jet-black liner. Her lids were greased and shaded, and her heavy brows, like Theda Bara's, curved in a downward arc. Her look was dangerous. These women—the early silent screen vamps—were the complete antithesis of the sweet-faced, wholesome heroines played by the Gish sisters, Mary Pickford, and Mabel Normand.

Any forward motion toward creative freedom for women came to a complete halt as the world prepared for war in Europe. The coming conflict, however, was a great class leveler. Shopgirls and duchesses, clerks and society dames, crossed class lines and pooled their time and resources, knitting socks and sweaters for the Doughboy and the British

Silent film star Pola Negri was a vamp, short for vampire—a film stereotype of a racy woman who used too much makeup and scent, wore blatantly revealing clothes, and was out to destroy man and family. Negri's eyebrows would look comical today, but in the 1920s they were all the rage.

Tommy, joining the nursing corps, and taking on jobs they'd never dreamed of for the war effort. Artifice and style took a backseat to patriotism and practicality. Corsets grew less restrictive and physically smaller; skirts got slimmer. Flowing tresses were cut to shoulder length and covered with nurse's caps or military kepis, or parted in the middle and held back by decorative velvet bands worn low over the forehead. During the war, the typical upper-class woman let her brows flourish like weeds. Her skin was pale, and one of her only concessions toward grooming was eyelids shined up with Vaseline.

If World War I interrupted the march of the emerging woman toward the cosmetics counter, the minute it was over, women couldn't get enough of the stuff. They bought what was available like it was going out of style. More and more products arrived on beauty counters daily.

In 1919, a nineteen-year-old named T. L. Williams watched as his sister Mabel sat at her dressing table, applying Vaseline to her lashes. In a flash of inspiration, young Williams was spurred to develop a product called Lash-Brow-Line, which he sold for a quarter. He named his company after his sister: Maybelline.

As the century grew older, women had proved themselves as useful citizens, they had maintained their femininity, and now they were up for some big fun. For inspiration, they turned to the movies.

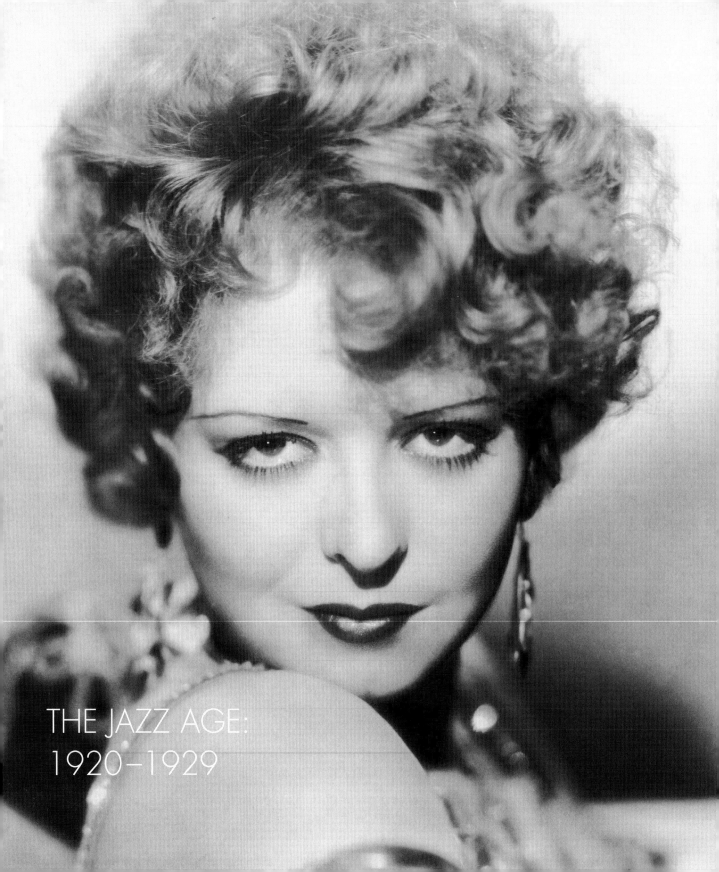

THE JAZZ AGE:
1920–1929

In 1920, two things happened: Women got the vote, and dancer Irene Castle cut her hair. The new style was called "the Chop." Short and saucy, it framed Castle's face, focusing ample attention on her eyes. Young girls embraced the hoydenish, boylike style, bobbing their hair and taking advantage of their newly elevated status to do as they pleased. The Roaring Twenties were upon them.

After the cataclysm of the First World War, the 1920s were a decade of devil-may-care. It was a full pardon for women, who consolidated their wartime gains. The stylish woman of the 1920s was young and ready for anything. By cutting her hair, she cut her ties to Victorian morality. With the new labor-saving devices (such as washing machines and indoor plumbing with hot water) and birth control, she took charge of her own life. She wore stockings rolled to her knees and bound her breasts to accommodate the sliplike chemise that hung from her shoulders and slid past her waist. On her cropped hair, she wore turbans or cloche hats that snuggled low over her eyebrows, often obscuring half her face.

Smaller-looking heads and shorter hair, shingled or marcelled into careful waves (a process invented by a Parisian hairdresser named Marcel Grateau at the turn of the century), required more exacting makeup on the eyes and brows. Women learned to

Clara Bow, the original It Girl, was the quintessential flapper, with teensy, flyaway brows, bee-stung lips, and a cropped mop of unruly curls.

take more time with their looks. Androgynous, adorable, and infused with an independent spirit, a woman's face reflected her new freedom, with bee-stung lips and superciliously tweezed brows that telegraphed her lack of concern for old moral codes.

Beauty was no longer considered a sin or a duty, but a creative pleasure. Silent film stars were the icon. Their faces, hair, lips, lashes, and brows set the styles for the girls with disposable income, curiosity, and more than a dollop of exhibitionism. They copied the looks they saw on screen and took them out into not-so-polite society.

Since the birth of the silent film era and the star system in 1911, a leading actress's face was her fortune. Her eyes spoke more loudly than the words you couldn't hear. Directors such as D. W. Griffith and Cecil B. DeMille used their cameras to exploit the emotional nuances of the human face, particularly the eyes which, in close-up, did all the heavy emotional lifting. Without the proper eyebrows, however, the eye lost its power. To make the area of expression even more focused, makeup artists cleared the field by paring down the brows. Mobile, emotive, tweezed eyebrows were more readily understood by the camera.

In her book *A Life on Film*, actress Mary Astor, whose career spanned both the silent and the talking film eras, describes her early film makeup ritual. Greasepaint was Stein's No. 2, powdered to masklike perfection. She wore no shadow but plenty of black mascara. The beaded effect was accomplished with

Comitique, a waxy, black substance that was melted over an oil lamp and applied singly to each lash with a toothpick.

A full ten years before the 1930s, when eyebrows nearly ceased to exist, screen star Clara Bow, dubbed the It Girl ("It" being sex appeal), tweezed her brows down to a skinny line that sagged over the outer corners of her eyes. With her bobbed hair, cupid's-bow mouth, and redrawn brows, she was a precursor to the glossy sophistication of Marlene Dietrich, Norma Shearer, Jean Harlow, and Carole Lombard. Bow's brows were a crude effort, at best, and they made her look worried and pensive amid the other contradictory elements of her face.

Max Factor and the Westmore Brothers were the Hollywood makeup geniuses who established the signature look of the stars. Factor worked on all the film beauties of the day, perfecting their images, particularly the Jazz Babies, who were usually cast as shopgirls who lucked out by snagging rich guys. These stars were the Million-Dollar Babies—Clara Bow, Joan Crawford (then known as Lucille Le Sueur), Laura La Plante, Billy Dove, Vilma Banky, and Gloria Swanson.

Bow and some of the other fresh, new Jazz Baby stars, like Mae Murray, Colleen Moore, and Louise Brooks, were quintessential flappers, those reckless and racy new girls who smoked, drank, stayed up all night dancing the Charleston, and were daring enough to adjust their makeup in public.

Under her China-girl bangs, Brooks was an unforgettable example. She drew her eyebrows in slanting lines toward the outside corners of her eyes and dressed her lashes in mascara. But there was a sad and unexpected vulnerability to her face that mitigated her raunchy image, one that was cemented when she appeared toward the end of the decade as Lulu, the doomed courtesan in a German production of *Pandora's Box*. Brooks's own lifestyle seemed to parallel that of the tragic Lulu. Racing at breakneck speed, Louise Brooks went from man to man, attempting a rakehell life. But her sad brows gave her away.

In 1920, Factor was asked to change Gloria Swanson's breathless ingenue visage into a more marketable look. He converted the frizzy-haired young player with the Kewpie-doll mouth into a sophisticated woman. Straightening her new bob, he shaded Swanson's heavy-lidded eyes with smoky color and oiled her lids, taking advantage of their come-hither potential. He manicured her brows into carved arches. No more were there to be primitive, angry, willy-nilly stabs of black above the brow. Overnight, Swanson became a soignée, sophisticated, thoroughly modern woman, replacing the fading Theda Bara as the new vamp.

But Swanson had some very steep competition. In 1925, Greta Garbo arrived in the United States from her native Sweden. She was sent directly to Factor for a "makeup dramatization" for her screen test. The makeover was to influence what western women would do to their faces for a decade. Factor arched Garbo's already beautiful brows and took out every hair but the essential ones. In doing so, he expanded the area from the lashline to the arch, where the cameraman could play with light and shadow. The combination of Garbo's thick lashes, hooded eyes, and uncompromising arch resonated with American women.

The Garbo eye, however, was not purely the invention of a Hollywood makeup man. In truth, the face that most actresses wore in the films of the 1920s was a copy of the British aristocrat's haughty visage that costume designers and makeup men saw in fashion magazines and copied. With their highly tweezed brows and their contoured cheeks (rouge was placed under the cheekbone, and brows were arched and plucked into a thin line), the women of the British ruling class looked the part—snobbish, arrogant, disdainful, and unreachable. Garbo's handlers co-opted the face for the sultry Swede, and five years later so did Marlene Dietrich with her carefully drawn lip, sensually oiled eyelid, and imperious brow.

At the same time that the Silent Screen Siren was making inroads into the fashion consciousness of the young American flapper, Paris was exerting its own influence. After the war, there was a tremendous mixing of cultures in Paris as émigrés arrived from Russia, Hungary, Spain, and America.

There was an affection for things exotic. Ballerinas like Anna Pavlova and Tamara Toumanova

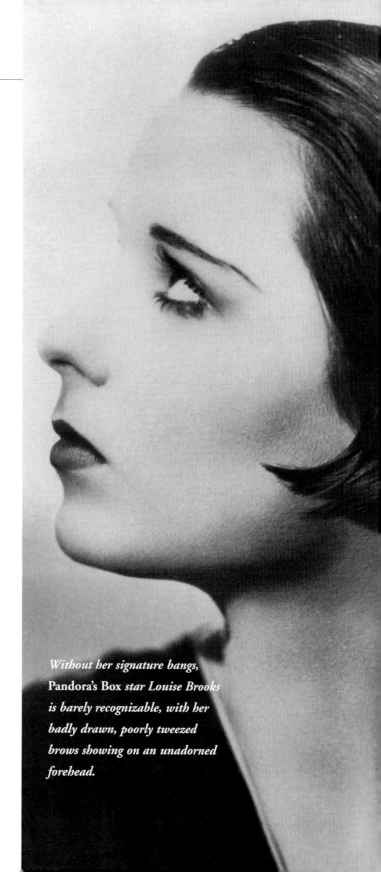

Without her signature bangs, **Pandora's Box** *star Louise Brooks is barely recognizable, with her badly drawn, poorly tweezed brows showing on an unadorned forehead.*

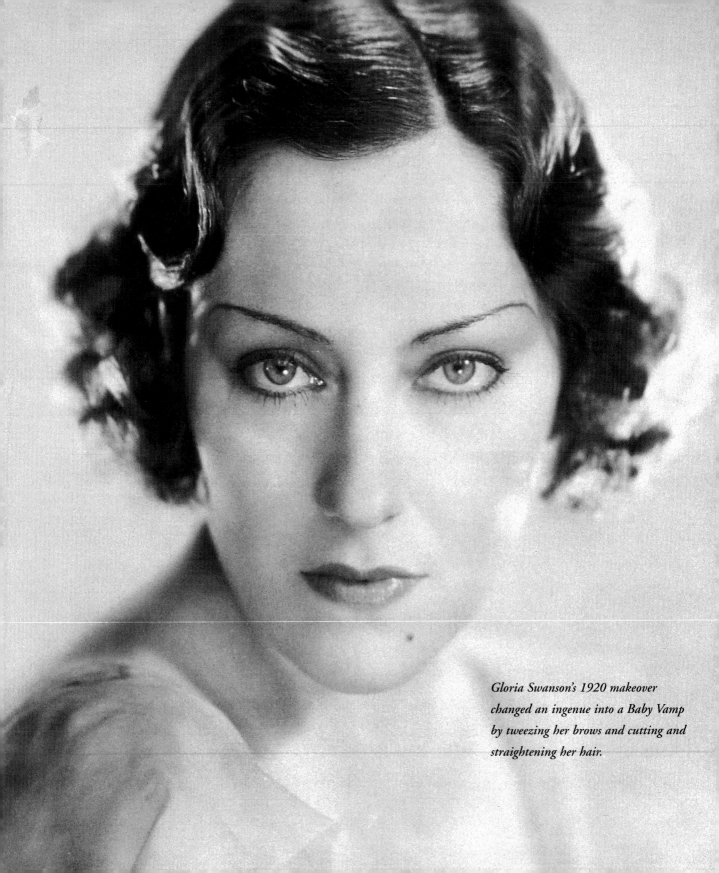

*Gloria Swanson's 1920 makeover
changed an ingenue into a Baby Vamp
by tweezing her brows and cutting and
straightening her hair.*

from the Ballets Russes wore stage makeup with slickly shadowed lids and beautifully defined, dark eyebrows that were clearly groomed and emphasized with a waxy pencil for an oiled look. In 1924, archaeologist Howard Carter opened the tomb of Tutenkhamen in Egypt, and soon Art Deco design was taking on the lines of artifacts found in the tomb. Onyx and diamond jewels from Cartier copied Egyptian motifs; chairs and chests were designed with lions' feet and hieroglyphics. The fad for dark eyes and even darker eyebrows continued.

The fascination with the exotic extended to the Far East, with the popularity of British silent star Anna May Wong, whose bangs, shiny brows, and almond-shaped eyes were replicated on Louise Brooks in *Pandora's Box* in 1928. Evening makeups were vivid and racy. Bright rouge was applied in doll-like circles and remained unblended. Eyes were shadowed in vivid colors or simply circled with heavy black lines for the exotic, Asian look. Brows were void of surplus hairs and were blackened with grease pencil. The artificial elegance of the French was celebrated in American *Vogue,* which set off another wave of women who copied the look.

Regardless of the influences, the cumulative beauty image of the 1920s was artificiality taken to a

Ballerina Alexandra Danilova's eye makeup, especially her eyebrows, was copied by women hungry for the popular exotic look of the 1920s.

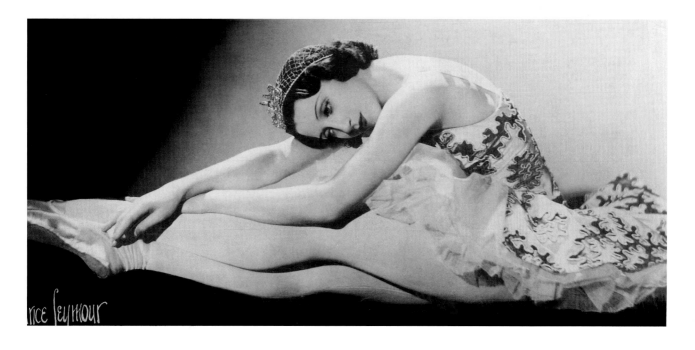

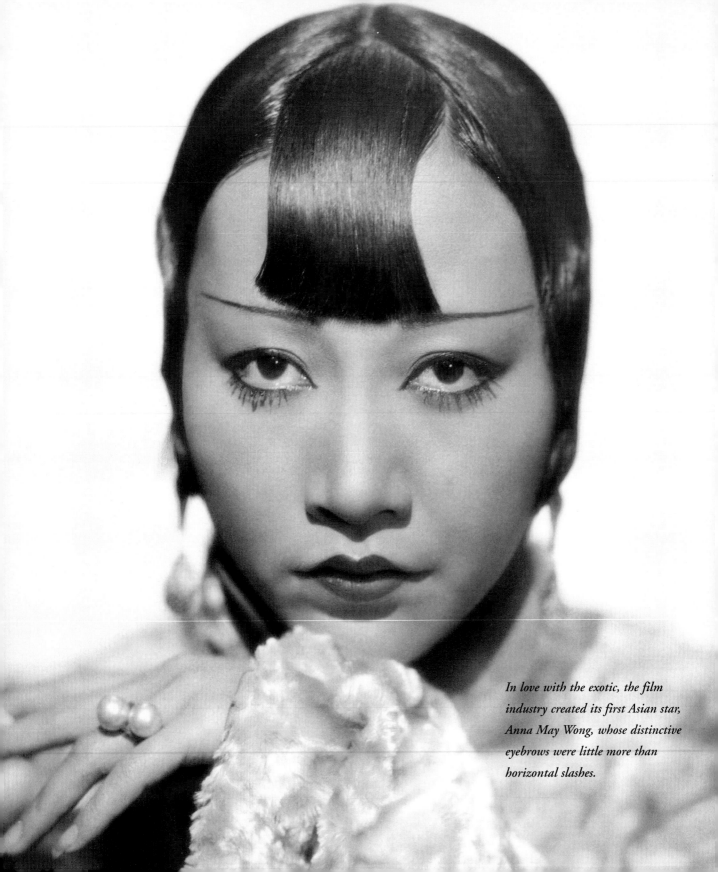

In love with the exotic, the film industry created its first Asian star, Anna May Wong, whose distinctive eyebrows were little more than horizontal slashes.

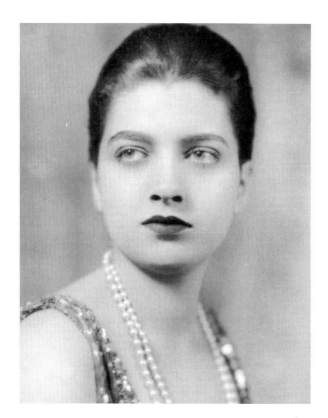

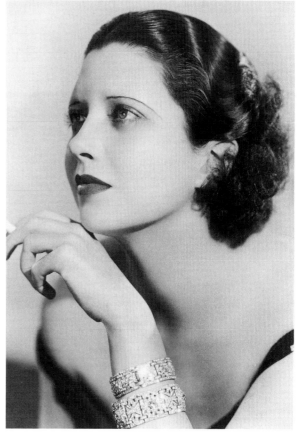

When Kay Francis arrived in Hollywood with her natural brows and full face, who would have thought that she would become a sophisticated, worldly comedienne with the polished, disdainful look that typified the 1930s?

By the time the stock market crashed on Black Tuesday, October 29, 1929, the world had fallen in love with Garbo, Dietrich, and a new baby wonder: Jean Harlow, the original Platinum Blonde.

high degree. Modern colors were as shocking as they were audacious. Turquoise and alarming poison green were favorite eye shadow hues. The doll-like circle of rouge made its way from Paris to the States. There was no subtlety or blending. Eye makeup was the most experimental aspect of the 1920s face. Cake, tube, wax, and liquid mascaras were advertised in magazines. Eyebrow pencils were limited to black and brown and were often used not only to enhance or obliterate the natural brow, but to dot the outside corner of the eye where the upper and lower lashes met to make the eye seem larger.

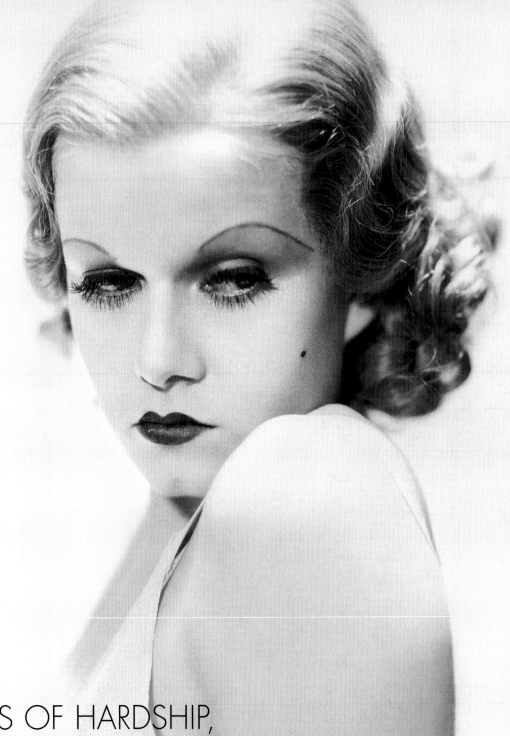

YEARS OF HARDSHIP,
YEARS OF GLAMOUR: 1930–1939

By the beginning of the 1930s, a woman's face had been manicured into artificial perfection. Film stars allowed their own features to become obscured and remade by makeup artists who overdrew their natural liplines and obliterated their eyebrows, only to redraw an idealized, graphic brow with black pencil. The brows, if they existed at all, were anemic and waiflike. They gave the face the appearance of perpetual surprise and irony.

The idealized faces of Jean Harlow, Marlene Dietrich, and Greta Garbo—so pristine in their flawlessness that they looked to be carved from purest white marble—hit the screen at the height of the Depression. The comedies of Preston Sturges and the fluffy frou-frou of Busby Berkeley's kaleidoscopic dance numbers in films like *42nd Street, Top Hat, Golddiggers of 1934*, and *The Ziegfield Follies* were light, frothy entertainments crafted by Hollywood to get people's minds off deprivation, soup kitchens, and unemployment lines.

The scatterbrained comedienne Carole Lombard, the twinkle-toed dancer Ginger Rogers, and the harlots with the hearts of gold, Jean Harlow and Mae West, were painted to a fare-thee-well with smooth complexions and gently mascaraed, barely lined eyes,

The original Blond Bombshell, Jean Harlow, looked more corn-fed than cat-sleek when she first arrived in town, but by 1930, with her platinum bob, Kewpie-doll mouth, and narrow tracery of drawn-on brows, a film goddess was born.

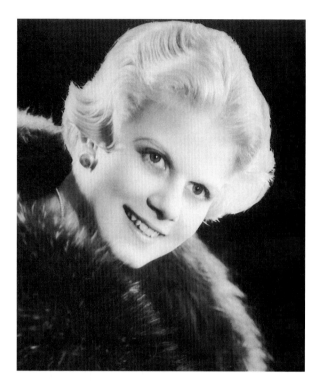

blinking out from under bitsy brows that were shaved or tweezed out and redrawn with architectural precision. There was nothing real about any of it.

The face of the Thirties was all drop-dead glamour. The Ideal took precedence over the Real. Stars telegraphed a richness and sophistication that probably only existed, in this time of financial hardship, in the minds and cameras of the Hollywood filmmakers. Attitudes about clothing and cosmetics, however, were changing. Some of this change was forced by the new film censor, the Hayes Office, and some of it was the natural swing of the pendulum back from the outrageous flapper look to a more refined appearance.

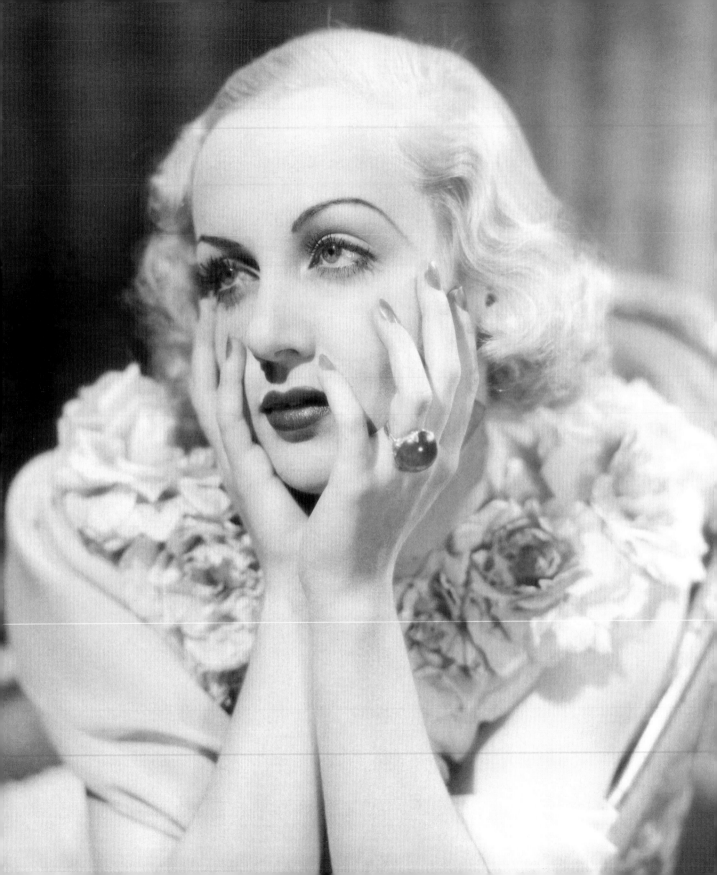

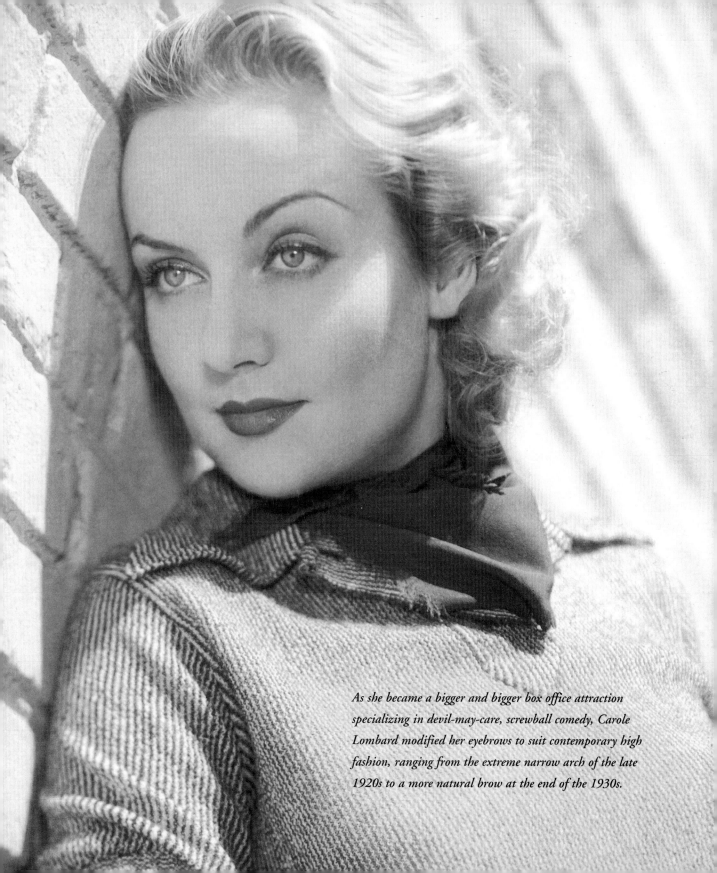

As she became a bigger and bigger box office attraction specializing in devil-may-care, screwball comedy, Carole Lombard modified her eyebrows to suit contemporary high fashion, ranging from the extreme narrow arch of the late 1920s to a more natural brow at the end of the 1930s.

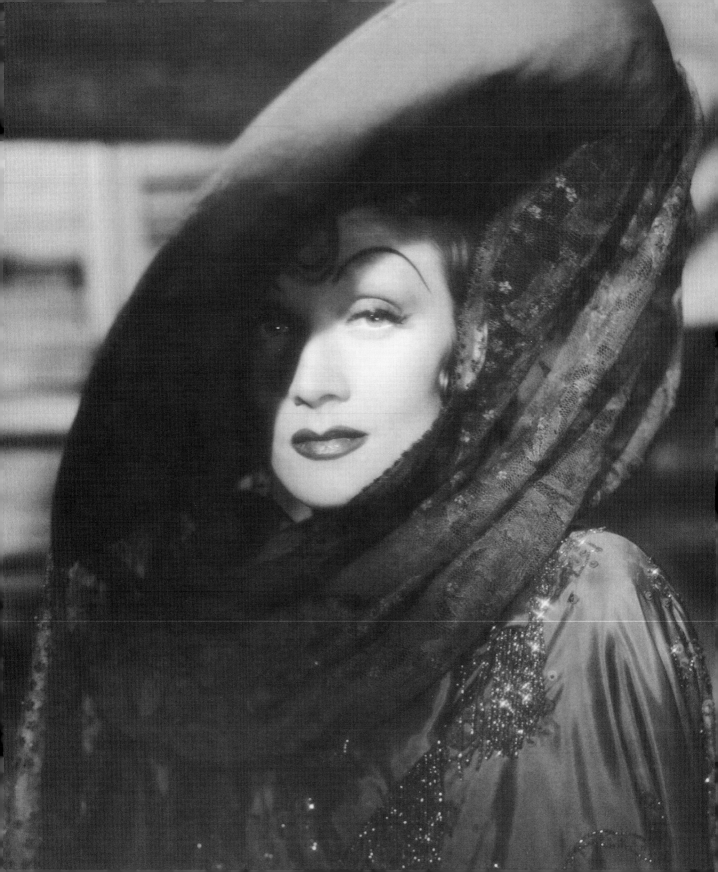

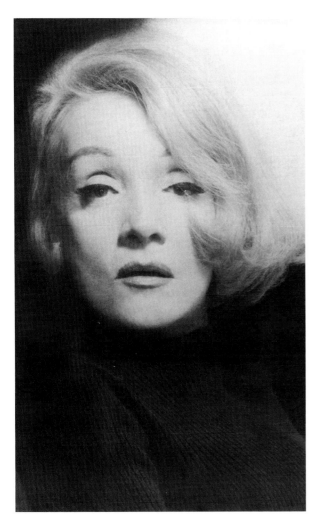

After she filmed The Blue Angel *in 1930, the German-born future Femme Fatale Marlene Dietrich completely remade her image. She tweezed her eyebrows so radically, studio makeup artists begged her to let them grow in. She refused, and an unforgettable icon was established. But a woman can change her mind, as Dietrich did toward the end of her career. Good thing they were able to grow back.*

Women of the 1930s were not out to shock, tease, or repel, but to attract and seduce through frosty perfection and enigma.

The Hayes Office dictated draconian changes in the amount of cleavage and frontal nudity a movie queen could show on screen. But costumers like Adrian created an even sexier image by putting actresses in silky, body-hugging, bias-cut satin gowns that revealed more in contour, drape, and outline than a low-cut dress ever would. These dresses, like elegant nightgowns, rose high in the front, revealing the outlines of breasts and nipples, and they dipped dangerously low in the back, displaying acres of white skin. To match this statuesque perfection, hair turned a platinum blond, especially when a high-resolution panchromatic black-and-white film was developed that could "read" the whiteness of the hair and not cause a glare (and not wash out the face either). For the new film, Max Factor developed his Panchromatic makeup. He decided to experiment with lightening his stars' hair with peroxide. The results showed up not only on Harlow, but on many of the starlets: Paulette Goddard, Alice Faye, Bette Davis (who was rumored to have hated her blond hair), Ida Lupino, and even the well-established Norma Shearer.

Film studios now had resident makeup artists, who treated stars' faces as if they were blank canvases. The sophisticated countenances peering out from the screen were objects of fantasy, of dreams come true. Even the poorest shopgirl, collecting empty soda bottles to cash in for the nickel it cost to get into the movies, could imagine that with the right paint and powder and the right eyebrow, she too could be glamorous. Stars like Harlow and Garbo, with their perfect faces and high-flown brows, prompted avid, fashion-forward females to pluck their brows into minuscule lines or shave them off altogether and redraw them with oily pencil so the light could catch the gleam.

Not since medieval maidens shaved off their brows had the eyebrow been so small. These brows, whispers of what they had once been, had the opposite effect of those of their medieval sisters. Instead of the virginal pureness of the perfect egg, the Thirties screen goddess wished for sculptural perfection and frosty sensuality.

The movies had popularized a face that was so carved and glossy, it didn't look real. Brows were plucked so thin, they looked like ant tightropes. Harlow's brows were miracles of brevity. They fit with Harlow's soft-hard knowingness of the slightly tarty Kewpie doll—a wisecracking, sassy, brassy broad who took very little seriously. Until her untimely death at the age of twenty-six from kidney failure, she presented a gay, devil-may-care face to her public.

Unlike Harlow, the foreign-born Dietrich and Garbo had a much sexier remove. Cool and aloof, Marlene Dietrich remade most of her own image from her film debut in the States as a pudgy femme fatale in *The Blue Angel*. Preferring to do her own makeup, Dietrich once showed the men of the

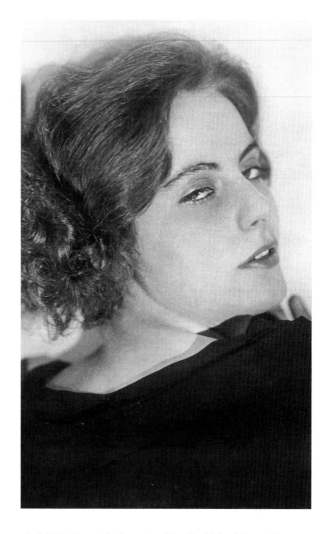

In 1925, Greta Garbo arrived in the United States from her native Sweden, and immediately film studio makeup artists worked their magic, turning a chunky charmer into a film goddess by paying close attention to her architectural bone structure. They slimmed her body, tinted her hair, and pared down her eyebrows to their elegant essence so that the allure of her eyes would blossom on-screen.

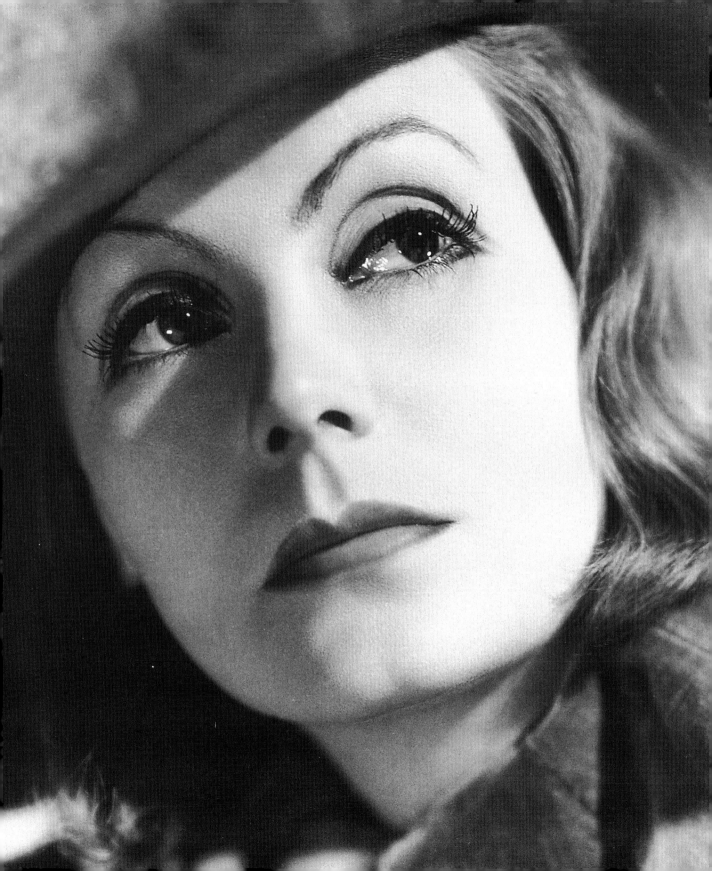

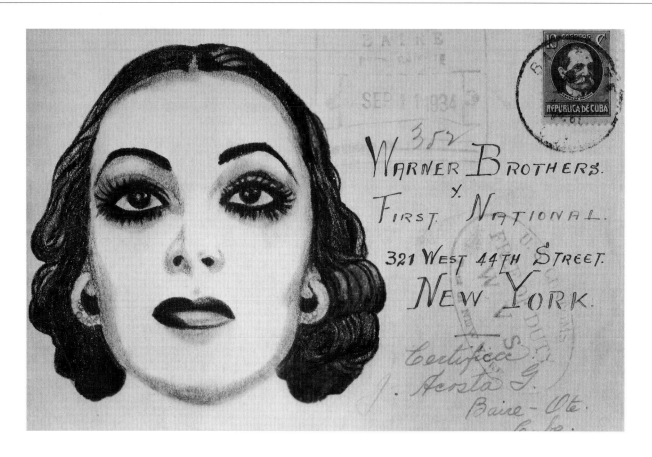

Cuban spitfire Dolores del Rio played up the dark exoticism of her eyes and eyebrows, as shown in this postcard from 1934.

Westmore makeup dynasty how she made eyeshadow. She burned a safety match under a white china saucer and mixed the resulting carbon with a few drops of baby oil, which she applied to her lids with the tip of her finger. As her brows got thinner and thinner, the Westmores and other studio makeup artists suggested that she had gone too far, that she should let them grow in a bit. But she resisted. She wanted deep-lidded

mystery, which she accomplished by accenting the outside corners of her own top lashes with a few well-placed fakes. They appeared to weight her eyes down to her alluring, come-hither visage: the sleepy, half-open, sexy sneer, punctuated at times by the trailing smoke of her cigarette.

Garbo's makeover, on the other hand, was purely the concoction of the studio system. Her mystery and sensuality flowed from lightly shadowed, Vaseline-coated lids, precisely mascaraed lashes, and ironically arched eyebrows. Was she as enigmatic and opaque as she seemed? Did the perfect arch of her brow represent ennui? Or was her face so gorgeous in repose that while she was thinking nothing, she presented the perfect, blank canvas on which the audience projected their own hopes and dreams? (It was probably the latter.)

When Garbo went through her studio redesign, Frederick Hall wrote in *Stage* magazine in 1934, "They smartened her up. They fixed her blonde hair, gave her a shape, and realizing that those eyes were

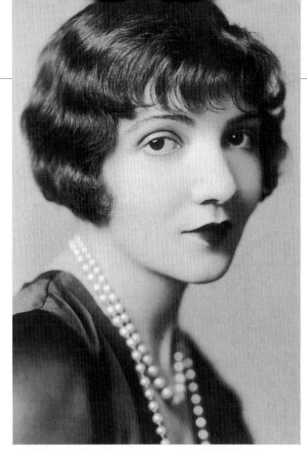

Claudette Colbert had signature bangs that fluttered perkily above eyebrows that followed the arc of contemporary fashion. She had a full set of natural brows in the early 1920s, but by the 1930s, makeup artist Monty Westmore tweezed them into a stylishly slim line.

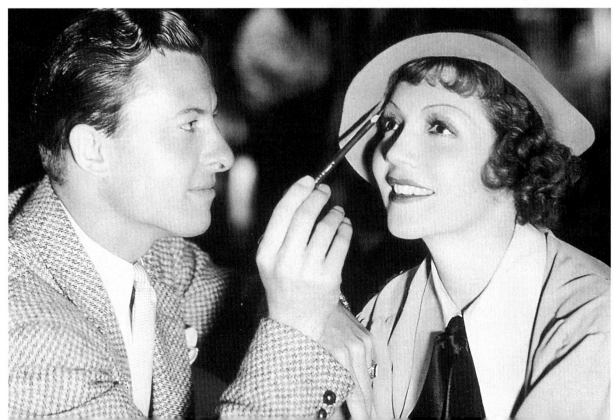

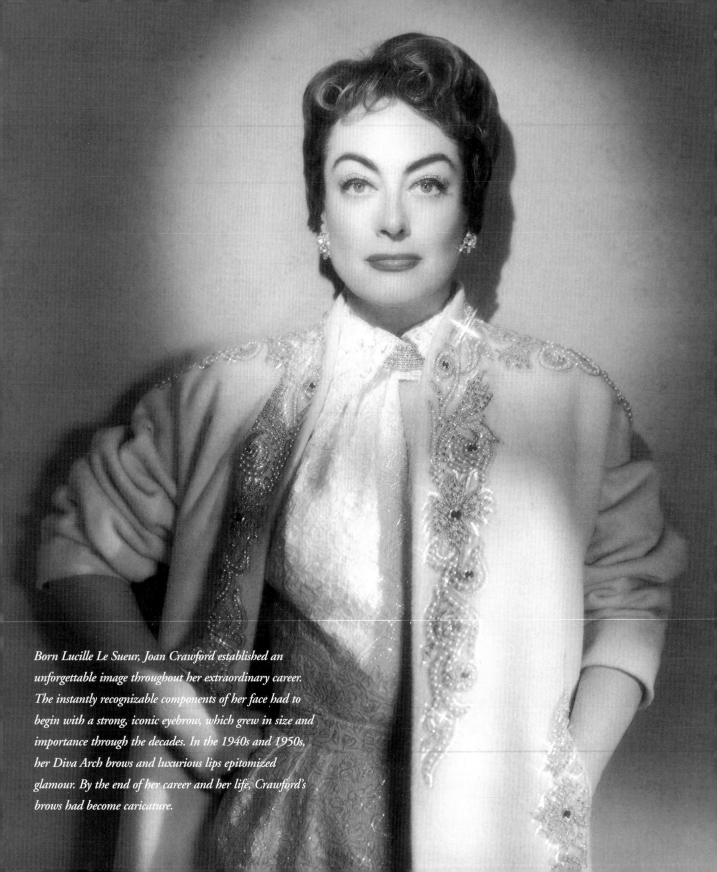

Born Lucille Le Sueur, Joan Crawford established an unforgettable image throughout her extraordinary career. The instantly recognizable components of her face had to begin with a strong, iconic eyebrow, which grew in size and importance through the decades. In the 1940s and 1950s, her Diva Arch brows and luxurious lips epitomized glamour. By the end of her career and her life, Crawford's brows had become caricature.

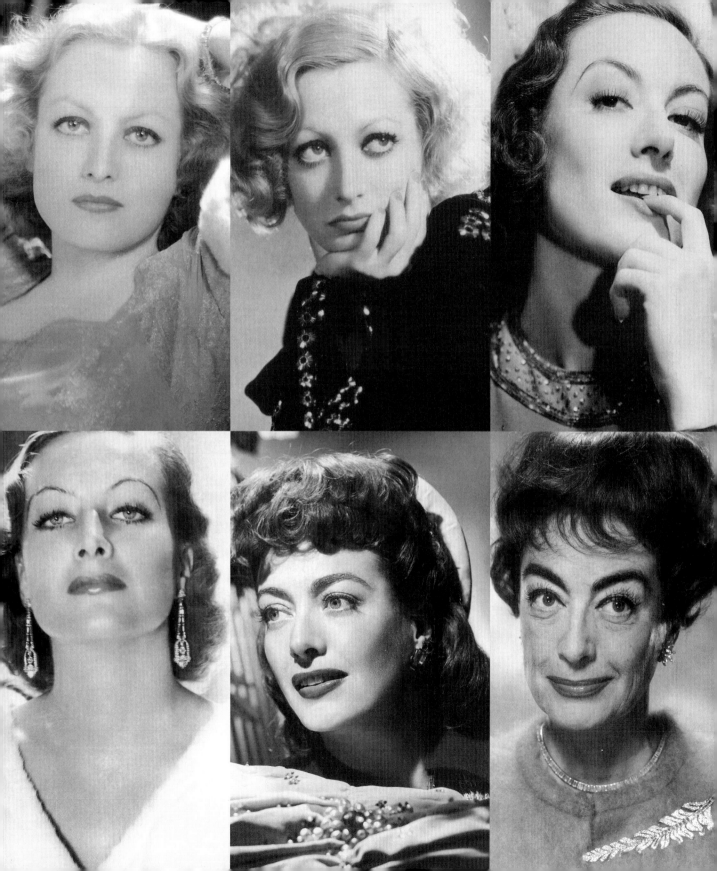

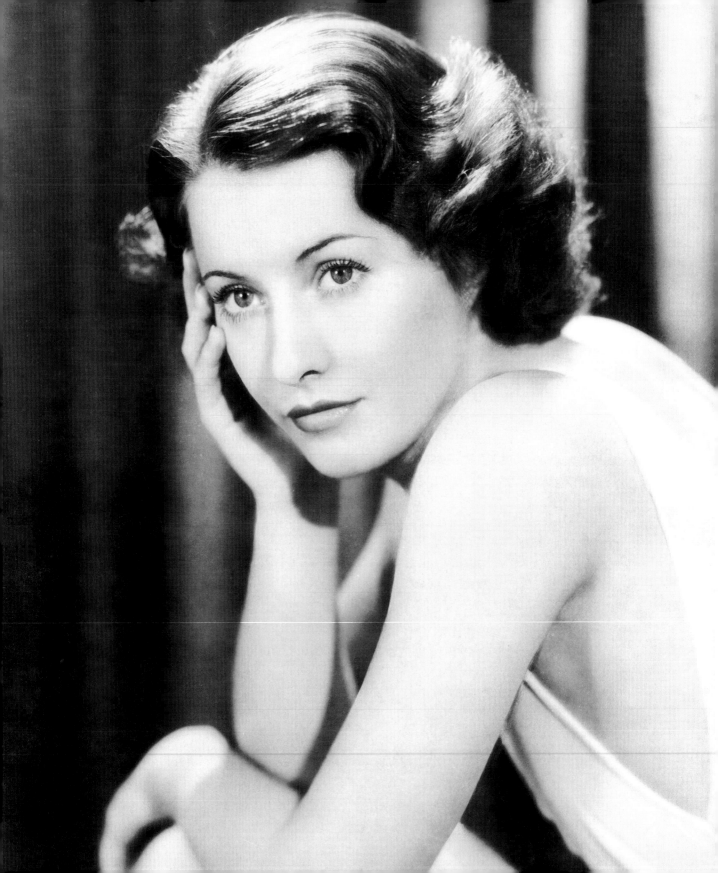

With her neatly formed brows and forthright gaze of the 1930s, Barbara Stanwyck's tough girl image could only be hinted at, with Double Indemnity *nearly ten years away.*

her finest feature, they made them up magnificently." Since 1929, she had been the biggest draw in Hollywood with that face and that "I want to be left alone" demeanor.

With a pair of eyebrows that were reduced to the essence of an arch, her face revealed features that were perfectly and ideally symmetrical, expressing every romantic emotion the camera needed to find.

Another actress who underwent a total metamorphosis in the 1930s was Joan Crawford. As a Twenties flapper and chorine, Crawford, known then as Lucille Le Sueur, had a bee-stung mouth and marcelled hair. In the mid–1930s, her features started to get bigger and bigger, and by late in the decade and into the early 1940s, her image was solidified: bossy brows and snarly lips. Her eyebrows were full, exaggerated, and overdrawn. They made a forceful statement and balanced her mouth, which had been outlined outside her own rather narrow lips and flared out at the corners. Crawford, it is said, often did her own makeup and refined her own look.

Stylistically, the Thirties appeared to be the all-white decade. White clothes. White rooms. (The decorator Elsie de Wolfe loved to design sparkling Art Deco rooms filled with snowy, white-upholstered furniture.) Fashion reflected those pristine surfaces— platinum hair, slinky white or cream satin dresses, and crisp, white ruffled collars and cuffs. High-definition photography displayed it all to almost surreal advantage. The studio still photographers manipulated light and shadow even more. In close-up portraiture by lensmen like Horst, Cecil Beaton, Hoyningen-Huene, Man Ray, and the impeccable George Hurrel, faces were perfect. Makeups were flawless. These studio portraits, published in the growing numbers of movie fan magazines, defined the look of the decade and promoted fans to duplicate it. Hurrel, who photographed the MGM stars, didn't let his subjects paint up too much. Often they came to his studio with just a thin layer of baby oil on their faces. The magical images came after the picture had been taken with his retouching art. More than anyone else, he created the look of actresses like Joan Crawford, Norma Shearer, and Claudette Colbert. No one knew, for instance, that Crawford was only five feet four and freckled from head to toe.

As the decade wore on, the look softened. Clothes became more filmy than slinky and were often well tailored, but the minimalist eyebrow stayed the same. Coco Chanel had adapted her lover Boy Capel's sporting attire for women—separates like cable-knit tennis sweaters, slim, ankle-length navy skirts, French-schoolgirl white collars and cuffs, and the exacting LBD, the little black dress. The divorcée Wallis Simpson, for whom Edward VIII abdicated his throne, was a study in prim chic. In her Molyneux

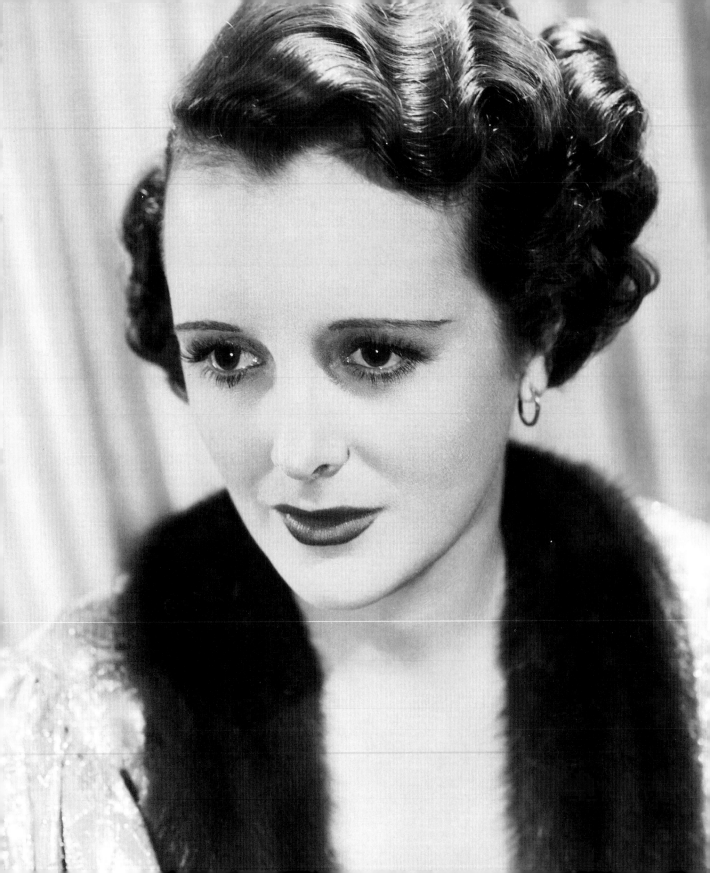

Mary Astor's career spanned the silent-to-the-talkies age,
and her eyebrows changed as makeup techniques improved.

and Mainbocher clothes, she had a straight, tight mouth and straight, tight brows to match.

As American *Vogue* chronicled the exploits and fashions of the society queens of the time, including Simpson and an assortment of Vanderbilts, Woodwards, and Whitneys, they declared: "Your eyelids and eyebrows should be shiny. Vaseline, gland cream, or brilliantine is very good for the purpose." At no time did they ever recommend that the brow be left alone or coaxed back into lush fullness. It took another world war and a new kind of celluloid stock to accomplish that feat.

With the development of Technicolor film, the thin, anorexic brow was on the way out. In 1935, *Becky Sharp* was photographed in full Technicolor. The film demanded much stronger lighting and yet another type of foundation. For black and white film, a face could be made flawless. With the correct lighting, the natural chiaroscuro of black and white could create a smooth, unblemished face.

Eyes could be made over, brows could be reshaped, and faces could be photographed to play up good bone structure.

But with Technicolor, movies demanded a far more natural look. Max Factor and his staff developed a nonreflecting makeup called Pan-Cake that read naturally. A solid cake makeup that was applied with a damp sponge, it proved to be so popular with actresses that they began stealing it from the studio. In one month, they swiped $2,000 worth. So, in 1938, the Factors—family patriarch Max had died in 1937—made a commercial version of it and called it Pancake Makeup—Pancake without the hyphen for the public.

As the world emerged from the depths of the Great Depression and prepared for war, one period of forced austerity was coming to an end, just as another was to begin. The first bona fide Eyebrow Decade of the twentieth century was coming to a close. The steely sexuality of Dietrich and Garbo and their thin, elegantly arched, sophisticated, nearly nonexistent brows were soon to be a memory as faint as their eyebrows.

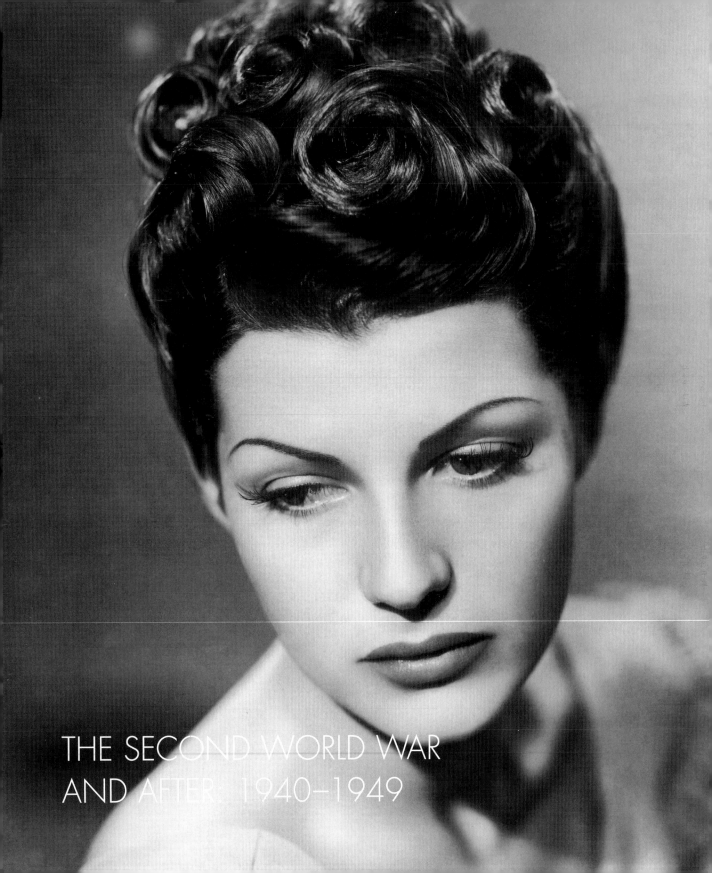

THE SECOND WORLD WAR
AND AFTER: 1940–1949

By the time the United States went to war after Pearl Harbor in December 1941, the American woman was a natural beauty. All the stylistic pretense and über-sophistication of the 1930s was gone, mostly because the patriotic woman simply didn't have time to fuss . . . nor did she have the cosmetics with which to do it. With the men away at war, women went to work as machinists, military drivers, radio operators, bus drivers, mechanics, and factory workers. With hair tucked safety under babushkas and into net bags called snoods, the new working women wielded wrenches and decreased their use of cosmetics to help the war effort.

Cosmetic production needed to be curtailed. So much of what went into lipstick and eyebrow pencils was strategic material—petroleum derivatives, glycerin, alcohol. Beauty products, however, were deemed essential to wartime morale, so some cosmetics, albeit quite dry, flaky, and unglamorous, were still on the market.

Companies like Yardley published morale-building messages in fashion magazines. Said one, "Never must careless grooming reflect a 'don't care' attitude. Now that leisure and beauty aids are limited, we must never forget that good looks and good morale are the closest of good companions. Put your best face forward."

Born Margarita Cansino, Rita Hayworth had a complete studio makeover before she hit it big in movies like Cover Girl *and* Gilda. *The makeover included electrolysis at her hairline and a redesign of her thick, beautifully constructed brows.*

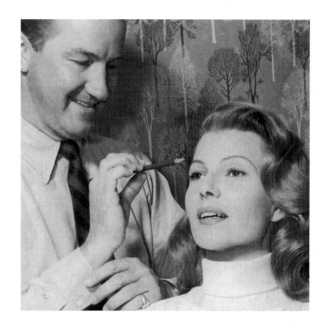

There was definitely a psychological value in looking good. Rosie the Riveter might have gone to work in body-obscuring coveralls and a tool belt, but she was wearing a swish of mascara and a dab of lipstick, and her brows were neatly tweezed and brushed on her all-American face. British *Vogue* admonished women: "You want [your beauty] to be a beauty that doesn't jar with the times, a beauty that is heart-lifting, not heart-breaking; a beauty that's beneficial, not glamorized; a beauty that's responsible—not a responsibility."

And so the marble statue–like perfection of the 1930s face gave way to a wholesome sexiness. Makeup was still scarce but available in limited quantities and considered a luxury, like sugar and beefsteak. Women let their high-maintenance brows go

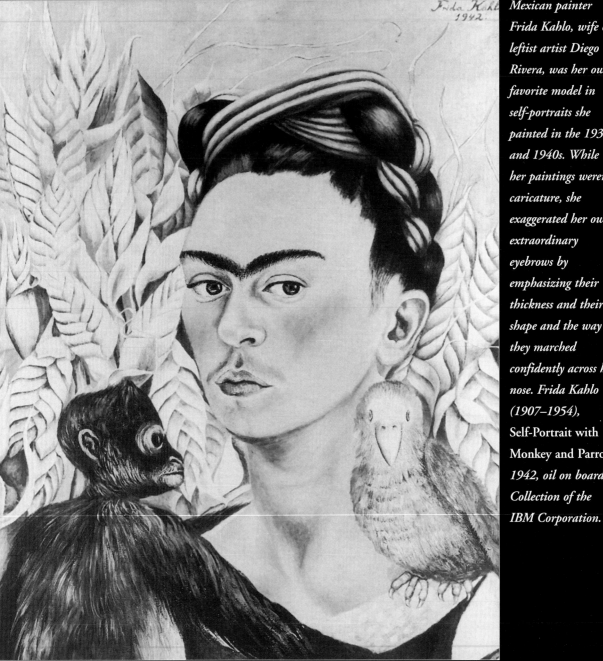

Mexican painter Frida Kahlo, wife of leftist artist Diego Rivera, was her own favorite model in self-portraits she painted in the 1930s and 1940s. While her paintings weren't caricature, she exaggerated her own extraordinary eyebrows by emphasizing their thickness and their shape and the way they marched confidently across her nose. Frida Kahlo (1907–1954), Self-Portrait with Monkey and Parrot, 1942, oil on board, Collection of the IBM Corporation.

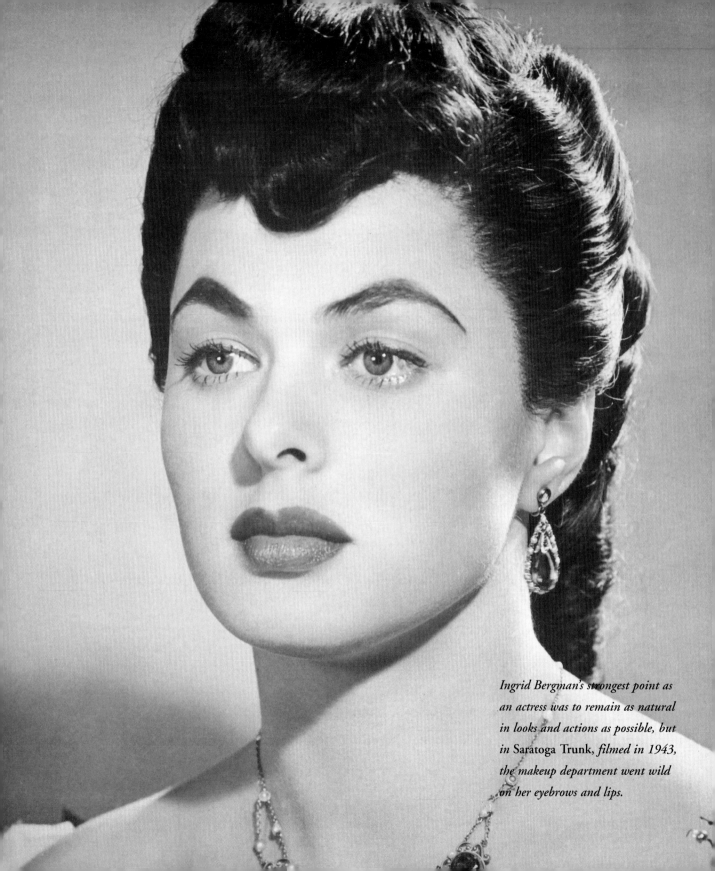

Ingrid Bergman's strongest point as an actress was to remain as natural in looks and actions as possible, but in Saratoga Trunk, filmed in 1943, the makeup department went wild on her eyebrows and lips.

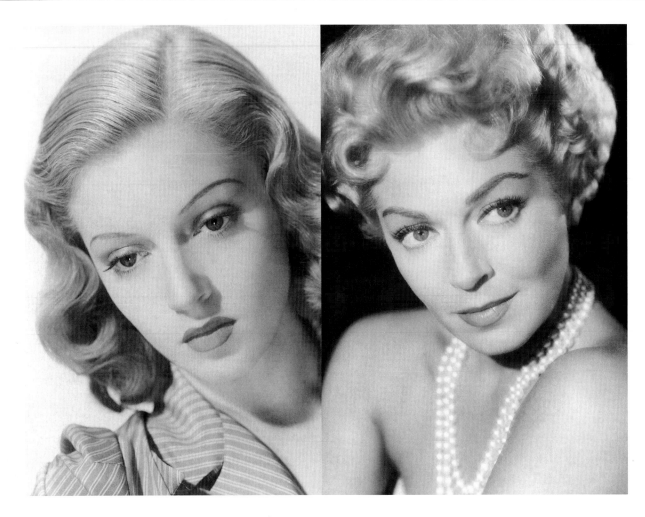

and instead used their eyebrow pencils as leg makeup (nylon and silk were strategic materials used for parachutes), drawing fake seams up the backs of their legs.

It was an inventive time. Or as *Vogue* put it: This was a time to "make do and mend." Oleo margarine was used as a cold cream substitute. British women used boot wax for mascara and shoe dye to darken their brows. In occupied

No, Lana Turner was not discovered sipping a soda at Schwab's drugstore, but studio heads knew they had a major glamour star and did her eyebrows accordingly through films like The Postman Always Rings Twice, The Bad and the Beautiful, *and* Imitation of Life.

France, soot and charcoal became eyeliner and brow blackener.

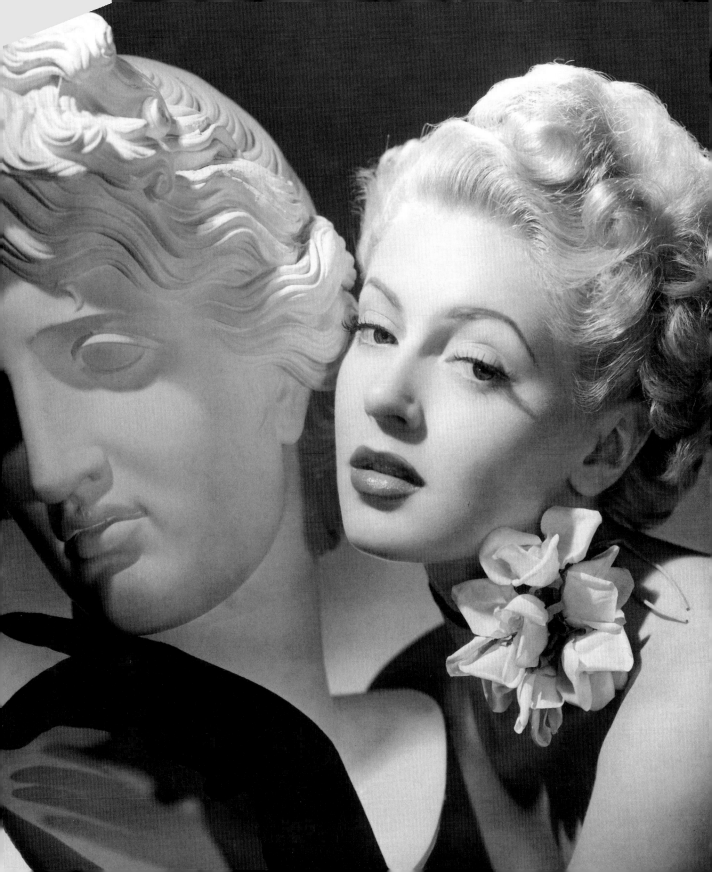

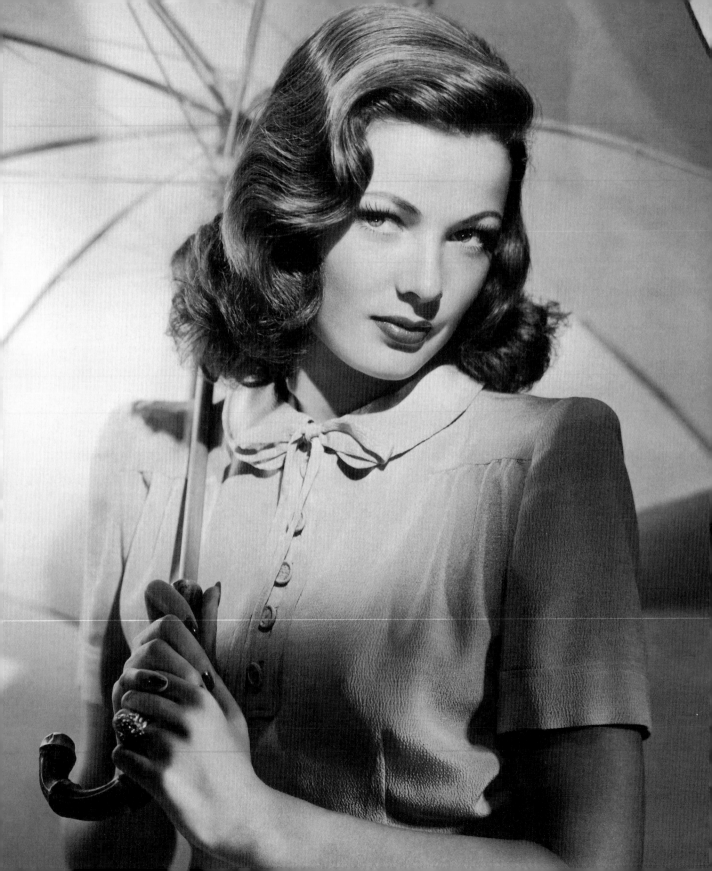

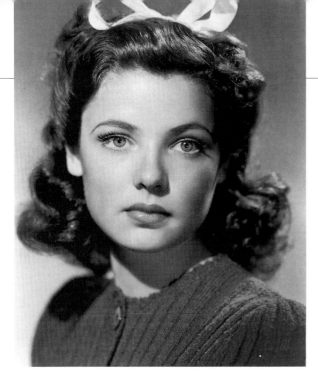

Possessor of the perfect natural arch, Gene Tierney and her graceful brows only got more beautiful and more patrician as they aged.

In Hollywood the soignée siren gave way to the wholesome pinup girl. Photographs of Betty Grable and her fabulous "gams" ended up in the lockers of soldiers, sailors, and marines in places as far away as Bastogne, Guam, and the Bulge. Ann Sheridan and Lana Turner were sexy, all-American sweater girls. And a whole new coterie of screen sirens emerged: Gene Tierney, Linda Darnell, Joan Crawford, Lauren Bacall, Rita Hayworth, Veronica Lake. Theirs was a more natural beauty, reinforced with elegantly coifed hair and strong brows.

Glamour in film was high drama. Crawford had her big shoulders, pouffy pompadour, thick brows, and exaggerated lips. Everything about her screen image was big, though in real life she wasn't. Lauren Bacall, the former fashion model who fell in love with and eventually married Humphrey Bogart, looked like a sultry college girl. In her 1944 test shots for *To Have and Have Not*, her hair was drawn up, pinned back, or worn down in a side-parted pageboy. All the styles held her hair away from her face, which put the focus on her heavy-lidded, gimlet eyes. Her eyebrows were distinctively tweezed. They dipped deep toward her nose with blunt, squared-off ends and soared high into a Diva Arch. It was a look that was to be prevalent in the 1950s, but Bacall had 'em first. Depending upon what she did with her brows, she could look haughty, angry, disdainful, or "touch at your own risk."

When the war ended and the men came home, women were suddenly relegated to their distaff jobs as housewives and mothers. While boyfriend and husband went to school on the G.I. Bill, the little "wifey" read her movie magazines and dreamed. Her whole fashion life received a massive jolt in 1947, when French couturier Christian Dior took advantage of the availability of cloth (for the first time in years, nylon, silk, wool, and cotton weren't rationed) and dropped the hemline down to midcalf.

Carmel Snow of *Harper's Bazaar* called Dior's wasp-waisted, Peter Pan–collared, crinolined skirted creations "the New Look." And it was. *Haute couture* was back with a vengeance, and cosmetics companies were just waiting in the wings to create *their* new look for *the* New Look.

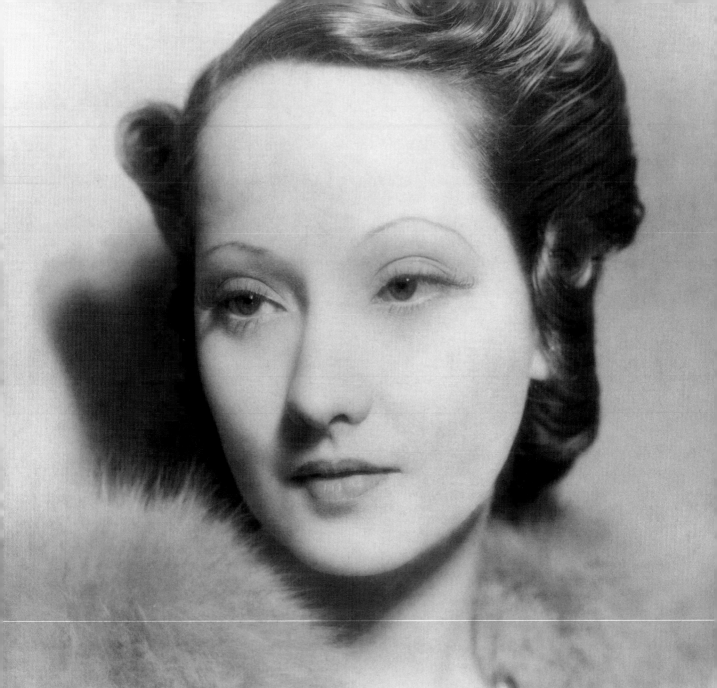

Exquisite in the 1930s, with her massively tweezed eyebrows, Merle Oberon evolved into a smoldering beauty whose redrawn brows, thick and luxuriant, balanced the perfection of her face.

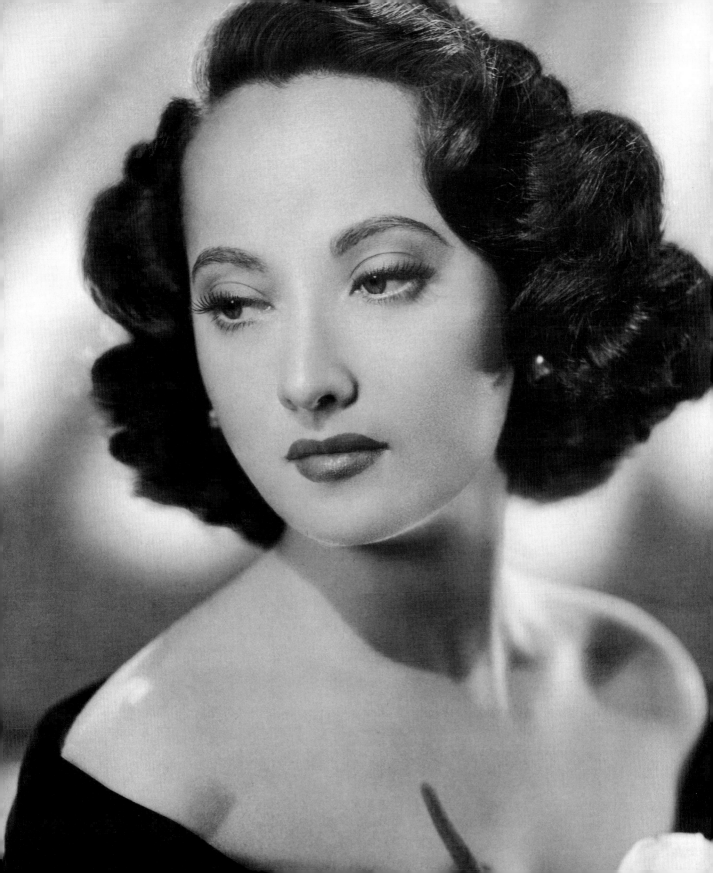

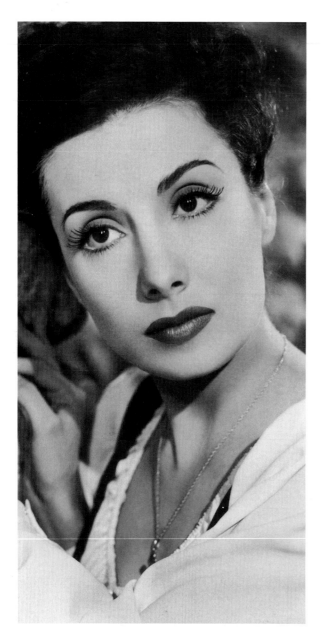

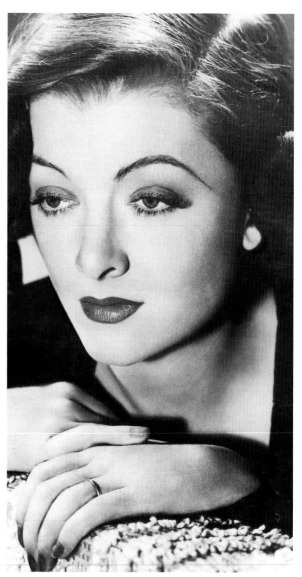

Myrna Loy, The Thin Man*'s Nora and society's darling, was the essence of classic sophistication, from her martini-dry repartee with costar William Powell to the clean and seemingly endless sweep of her eyebrows.*

Russian-born prima ballerina Tamara Toumanova starred with the America Ballet Theatre in the early 1940s.

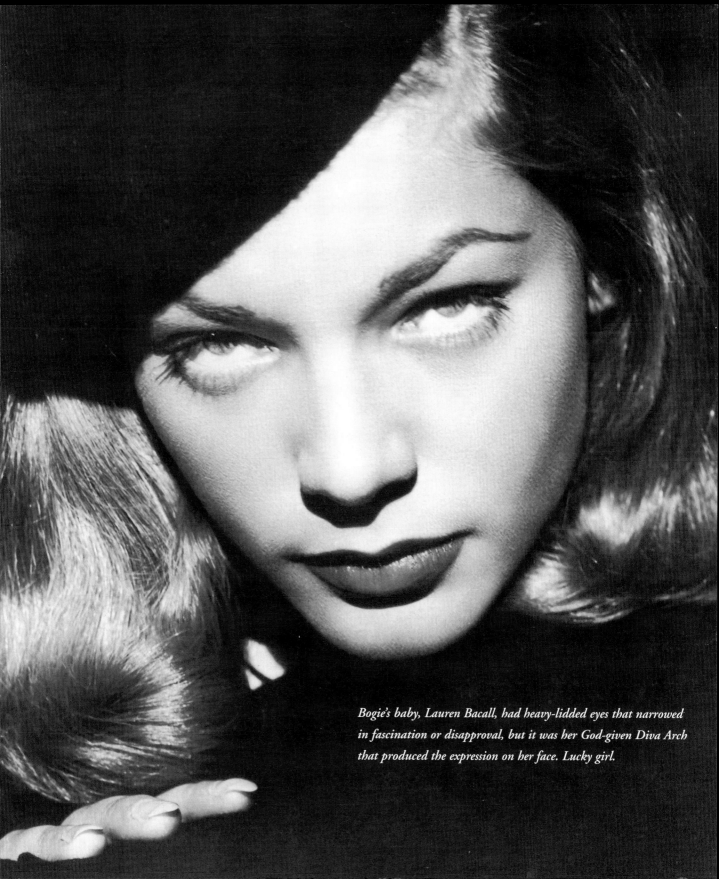

Bogie's baby, Lauren Bacall, had heavy-lidded eyes that narrowed in fascination or disapproval, but it was her God-given Diva Arch that produced the expression on her face. Lucky girl.

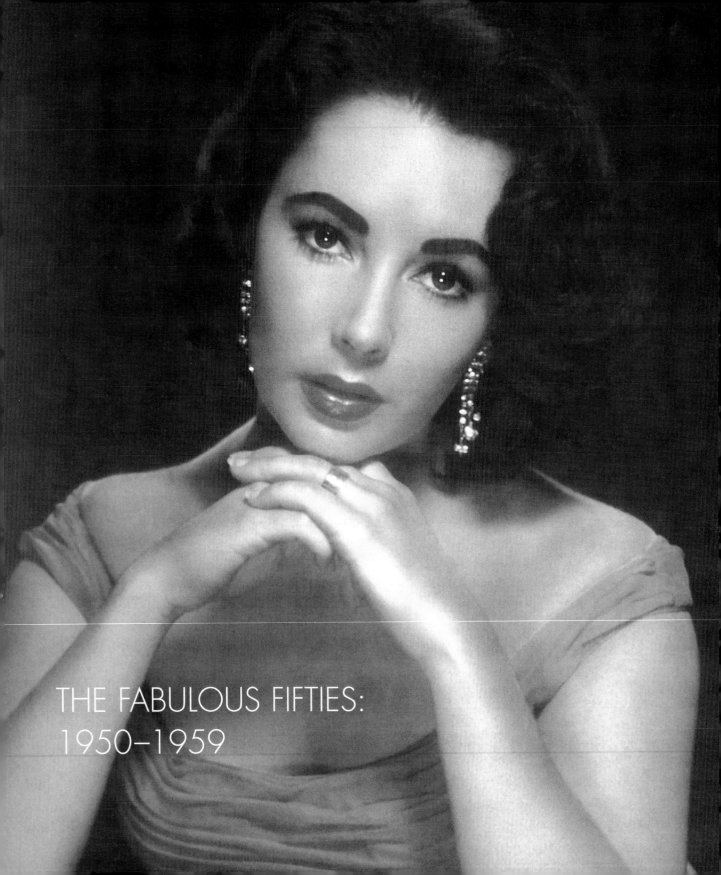

THE FABULOUS FIFTIES:
1950–1959

I f ever there was a decade dedicated to the worship and beautification of the eyebrow, it was the Fifties. Never has the brow had as much attention in all of its flagrantly full, expressive glory.

The face of the Fifties was as *haute* as the couture coming out of Paris. When Christian Dior declared that hemlines should swoop to midcalf, in a complete reaction to the shorter, tighter skirts and trousers of the 1940s, makeup had to respond. The New Look mirrored the international desire for extravagance and opulence after all the rationing and privation during the war years. The result was an era of elegance and sophistication that produced a strong image that is still instantly recognizable today.

Under Dior's creative eye, skirts were fluffed out with three or four horsehair crinolines. Not since the turn of the century had the body been so controlled and defined in figure-flattering but restrictive undergarments. The midsection was once again under the tutelage of the corset, this time called the "Merry Widow," which pushed the breasts up and out, exaggerating the bustline under the curvy femininity of Dior's hourglass shape. The rear end and thighs were encased in elastic panty girdles so that the butt would look flat and boy-slim under the calf-length sheath dress. The latter also came into fashion along with pointy-toed, three-and-a-half-inch stiletto-heeled shoes and wide, waist-cinching belts. The casual wardrobe was just as graphic a shape: skinny Capri pants, an untucked, white, man's shirt with the collar flipped up, and ballerina flats.

The New Look was a graceful, totally feminine fashion that bespoke the big-city chic of Paris and New York, which required an equally strong face. A woman had to *wear* her clothes, not the other way around. To support the drop-dead chic, the face had to be perfect. Not an extra, offending hair was allowed to sprout as brows arched into exaggerated grace. Even the hottest beauties had a cool edge.

The face of the Fifties had attitude to spare: brows arched in ironic amusement and lips colored the vampiest shades of red, fuchsia, and bright pink. It was a face to launch a thousand questions: Was she disapproving? Was she a tease? Is she amused? Is she *available*? If anything, the whole package—the *haute-couture* lines of her clothes and the graphic strength of her makeup—reinforced the Virgin Queen aspect of Fifties morality. A man had to marry the girl to see what was underneath her shapely but voluminous clothing. He had to give her the ring before she washed her face. In other words: The look of the Fifties was not user-friendly, intimate, or even fetching. It was as daunting to the woman who wore it as it was to the man or boy who courted her. But it was, and still is, totally memorable.

The most important component of the Fabulous Fifties face was the Diva Arch—an eyebrow so totally designed that it could carry the graphic eye that sat beneath it. The eyebrow was cultivated, pampered, and manicured into a soaring arch that peaked over the exact center of the iris. It was an amused arch, an ironic arch, but mostly, it

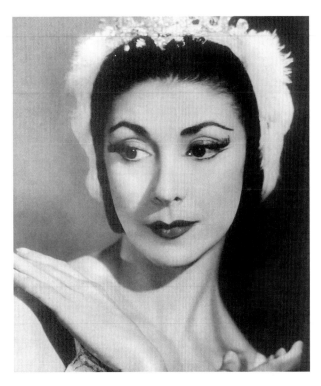

Dame Margot Fonteyn danced Swan Lake *in 1957, and her makeup was so copied by contemporary fashion, she may have felt at home on the street.*

was full, generous, and considered a statement of feminine perfection. But the whole face had to be perfect, too, especially the eye and the lip.

The shape of the 1950s eye came mainly out of Paris and from the ballet tradition that involved *l'oeil de biche,* the doe eye, which was designed by a Parisian makeup artist named Etienne Aubrey and featured prominently in American fashion magazines and on Hollywood's movie goddesses. Patently artificial and unnatural, the eye was overdrawn with a pre-

cise, thick, black line above the lashes that extended upward and outward into a wing at the end of the eye. Either the brow mirrored the shape of the eye, or vice versa. As for the lip, it was anything but neutral. (Somehow, toward the end of the century, contemporary makeup artists declared that a woman should choose between a strong eye and an obvious mouth. In the 1950s, she was allowed to have both.)

Women were getting their fashion information from several reliable sources—movies and magazines. Fashion magazines like *Vogue* and *Harper's Bazaar* covered designers such as Dior, Jacques Fath, Nina Ricci, Cristobal Balenciaga, and Pierre Balmain, who were doing their own versions of Dior's New Look; they also featured diagrams for proper eye makeup application and brow shaping. Women also read *Life,* which occasionally featured huge close-up portraits of film stars or fashion models on its glossy covers.

If Dior's more formal, shapely innovations promoted anything, it was the ascendance of the fashion photographer and magnificently groomed model-muse. The photographs of artists such as Richard Avedon, who posed Dovima in a magnificent ballgown against a massive elephant, could solidify a mood or an iconic look. Fashion photographer and portraitist Irving Penn photographed his wife, the radiantly aloof Lisa Fonssagrieves, whose face—with its dramatically swaggering, proudly arched brows—became the Look of the Fifties.

Another Fabulous Fifties face was that of Jean

Patchett, a major model of the period, whom *Vogue* used as its cover model in January 1950, to announce the arrival of *l'oeil de biche*. Patchett was a generically pretty brunette made special only by her extraordinarily forthright blue eyes. Her brows swooped over her eyes in perfect symmetry, with a high arch placed directly over the center of her iris.

Although Barbie wasn't a living doll, she was truly a Fifties invention. Twelve inches high, she had a bust that was so out of proportion that had she been a real girl she would have needed a tripod to hold her-

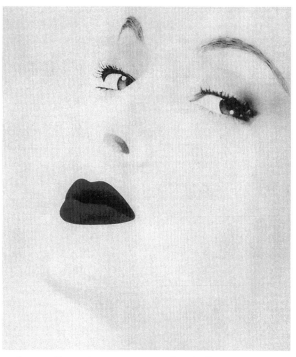

Where Hollywood stars once were the sole determining influences for the looks their adoring public would adopt, in the 1950s, models like Jean Patchett wore the look everyone copied: doe eyes and expressive brows with the exaggerated Diva Arch.

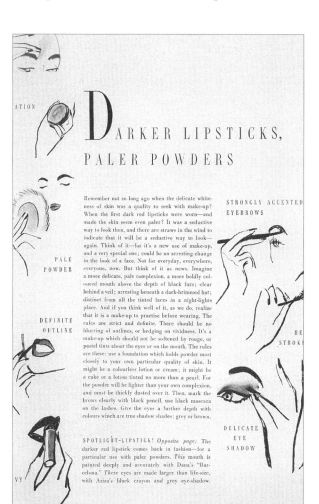

DARKER LIPSTICKS, PALER POWDERS

STRONGLY ACCENTED EYEBROWS

Remember not so long ago when the delicate whiteness of skin was a quality to seek with make-up? When the first dark red lipsticks were worn—and made the skin seem even paler? It was a seductive way to look then, and there are straws in the wind to indicate that it will be a seductive way to look—again. Think of it—for it's a new use of make-up, and a very special one; could be an arresting change in the look of a face. Not for everyday, everywhere, everyone, now. But think of it as news. Imagine a more delicate, pale complexion, a more boldly coloured mouth above the depth of black furs; clear behind a veil; arresting beneath a dark-brimmed hat; distinct from all the tinted faces in a night-lights place. And if you think well of it, as we do, realize that it is a make-up to practise before wearing. The rules are strict and definite. There should be no blurring of outlines, or hedging on vividness. It's a make-up which should not be softened by rouge, or pastel tints about the eyes or on the mouth. The rules are these: use a foundation which holds powder most closely to your own particular quality of skin. It might be a colourless lotion or cream; it might be a cake or a lotion tinted no more than a pearl. For the powder will be lighter than your own complexion, and must be thickly dusted over it. Then, mark the brows clearly with black pencil, use black mascara on the lashes. Give the eyes a further depth with colours which are true shadow shades: grey or brown.

SPOTLIGHT-LIPSTICK! *Opposite page:* The darker red lipstick comes back in fashion—for a particular use with paler powders. *This* mouth is painted deeply and accurately with Dana's "Barcelona." *These* eyes are made larger than life-size, with Aziza's black crayon and grey eye-shadow.

PALE POWDER

DEFINITE OUTLINE

HE STROK

DELICATE EYE SHADOW

self up. The Barbie doll was developed in 1958 by Ruth Handler who, with her husband, started Mattel Toys. The first Barbie had a ponytail, pouty pink lips, and the doe eye, but inexplicably, her brows belonged to the Thirties. They were mere painted wisps, set far too high on her elongated face to provide a role

Vogue taught its avid readers how to create high-fashion eyebrows at home in the November 1950 issue.

75

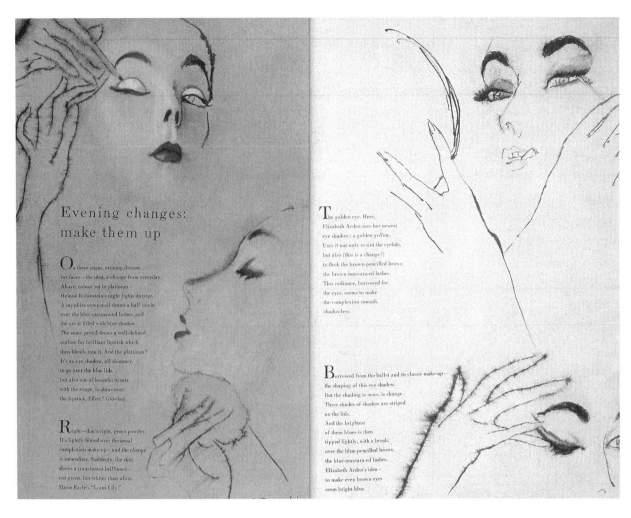

Evening changes:
make them up

On these pages, evening dresses
for faces—the idea, a change from everyday.
Above, colour set in platinum:
Helena Rubinstein's night lights dazzler.
A sapphire eye-pencil draws a half circle
over the blue-mascara-ed lashes, and
the arc is filled with blue shadow.
The same pencil draws a well-defined
outline for brilliant lipstick which
then blends into it. And the platinum?
It's an eye shadow, all shimmer,
to go over the blue lids,
but also out-of-bounds: to mix
with the rouge, to shine over
the lipstick. Effect? Glowing.

Right—that's right, green powder.
It's lightly filmed over the usual
complexion make-up—and the change
is immediate. Suddenly, the skin
shows a translucent brilliance—
not green, but whiter than white.
Marie Earle's "Lotus Lily."

The golden eye. Here,
Elizabeth Arden uses her newest
eye shadow: a golden yellow.
Uses it not only to tint the eyelids,
but also (this is a change!)
to fleck the brown-pencilled brows,
the brown-mascara-ed lashes.
This radiance, borrowed for
the eyes, seems to make
the complexion smooth,
shadowless.

Borrowed from the ballet and its classic make-up:
the shaping of this eye shadow.
But the shading is news, is change.
Three shades of shadow are striped
on the lids.
And the brightest
of these blues is then
tipped lightly, with a brush,
over the blue-pencilled brows,
the blue-mascara-ed lashes.
Elizabeth Arden's idea—
to make even brown eyes
seem bright blue.

An instruction sheet from the February 1955 Vogue.

model for the little girls who spent hours dressing and undressing her. Finally, in 1964, Mattel made her over to look like a wide-eyed California surfer girl, with long, combable blond hair and light, natural brows that extended the entire length of the eye.

Teenagers, meanwhile, were copying what they saw on-screen. With their hair cut in the fluffy "artichoke" style popularized by Gina Lollobrigida or the pixie cut seen on dancer Leslie Caron, all their attention focused on the eyes. While they traded in their orangey Tangee Natural and pinky-white, cherry-scented Milkmaid lipsticks for deeper Revlon colors such as Cherries in the Snow and Love That Red, they spent most of their time

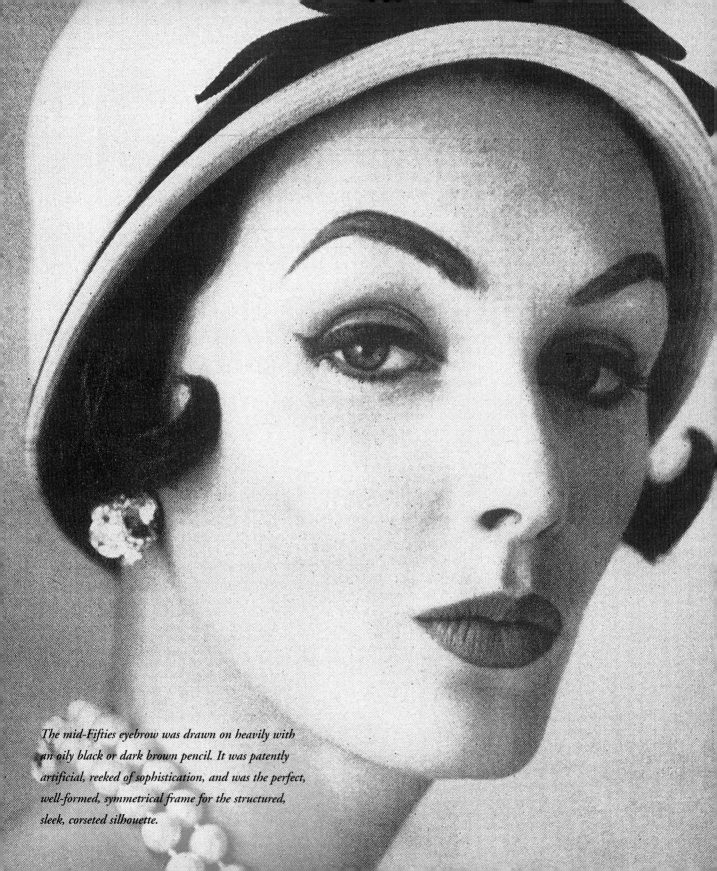

*The mid-Fifties eyebrow was drawn on heavily with
an oily black or dark brown pencil. It was patently
artificial, reeked of sophistication, and was the perfect,
well-formed, symmetrical frame for the structured,
sleek, corseted silhouette.*

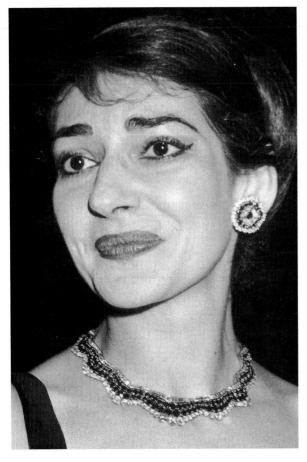

The diva with the Diva Arch: dramatic soprano Maria Callas at the height of her fame in the late 1950s

painstakingly lining their eyes with Maybelline cake mascara wetted down with saliva and stroked on with a tiny sable brush into bat-winged perfection. Carbon copies of their mothers, they wore cashmere twin sets in pastel colors, fake white collars called "dickeys," golden circle pins, and single strands of cultured pearls.

Hollywood, in the meantime, had not yet been co-opted by television and was turning out glorious Technicolor musicals, moody *film noir* thrillers, and domestic dramas. Actresses broke down into four definitive types: the Siren, the Blond Bombshell, the Girl Next Door, and the Gamine, but each of them, regardless of her typecasting, had one thing in common: the strong, graphic eyebrow.

Since the 1910s, screen sirens had been a staple of American film, and the goddesses of the 1940s consolidated their gains and polished their look in the 1950s—actresses like Joan Crawford, Bette Davis, Hedy Lamarr, Lana Turner, and Gene Tierney. The new generation of drop-dead glamour girls included newcomers like Ava Gardner, Gloria Grahame, and a young and breathtaking Elizabeth Taylor.

By the beginning of the 1950s, Crawford had honed her signature look to perfection. With her magnificent, thick eyebrows and her huge, over-drawn mouth, she was the personification of the bitch-goddess in films like *Torch Song, Sudden Fear, Autumn Leaves,* and *Johnny Guitar.* No victim she. Her face said it all. But it was her eyebrows that did most of the talking.

It was to be expected that brunette film stars have exquisite brows, because the raw material was already there with their dark hair. Elizabeth Taylor had been a child star at MGM, and even at age nine in *Jane Eyre* and at thirteen in *National Velvet,* her singular beauty was astonishing. But in the 1950s, when she made the transition from baby face to

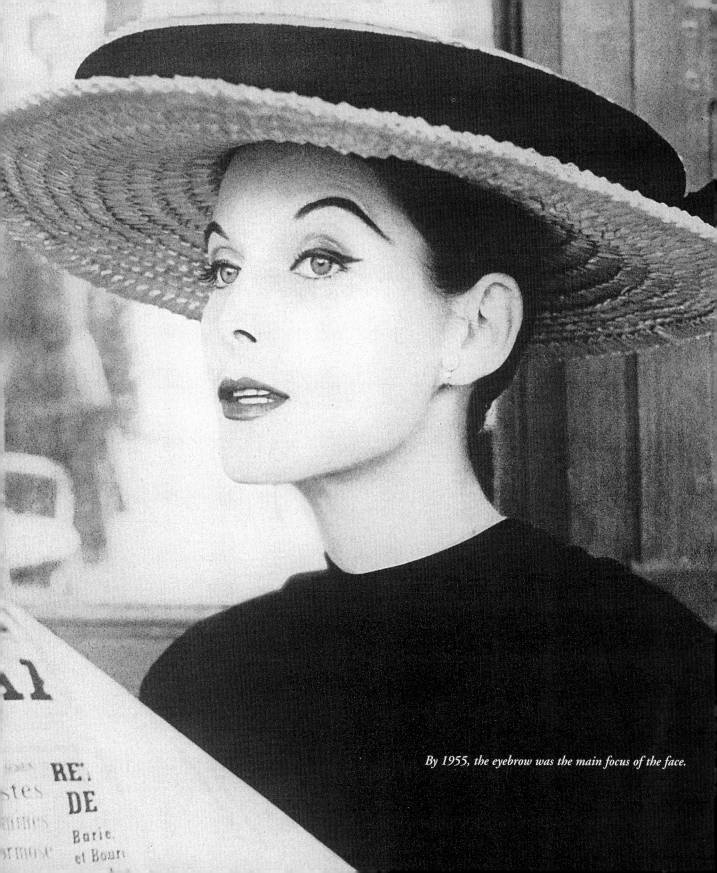

By 1955, the eyebrow was the main focus of the face.

VOGUE

c

ANUARY 15

Remaking
Yourself

NEW WAYS TO
Remake your figure's age...

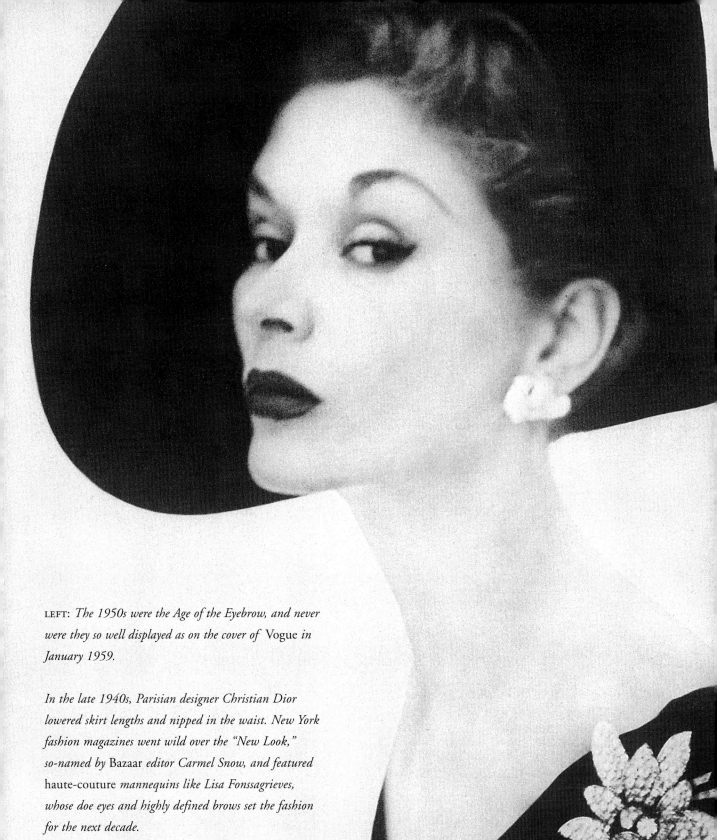

LEFT: *The 1950s were the Age of the Eyebrow, and never were they so well displayed as on the cover of* Vogue *in January 1959.*

In the late 1940s, Parisian designer Christian Dior lowered skirt lengths and nipped in the waist. New York fashion magazines went wild over the "New Look," so-named by Bazaar *editor Carmel Snow, and featured haute-couture mannequins like Lisa Fonssagrieves, whose doe eyes and highly defined brows set the fashion for the next decade.*

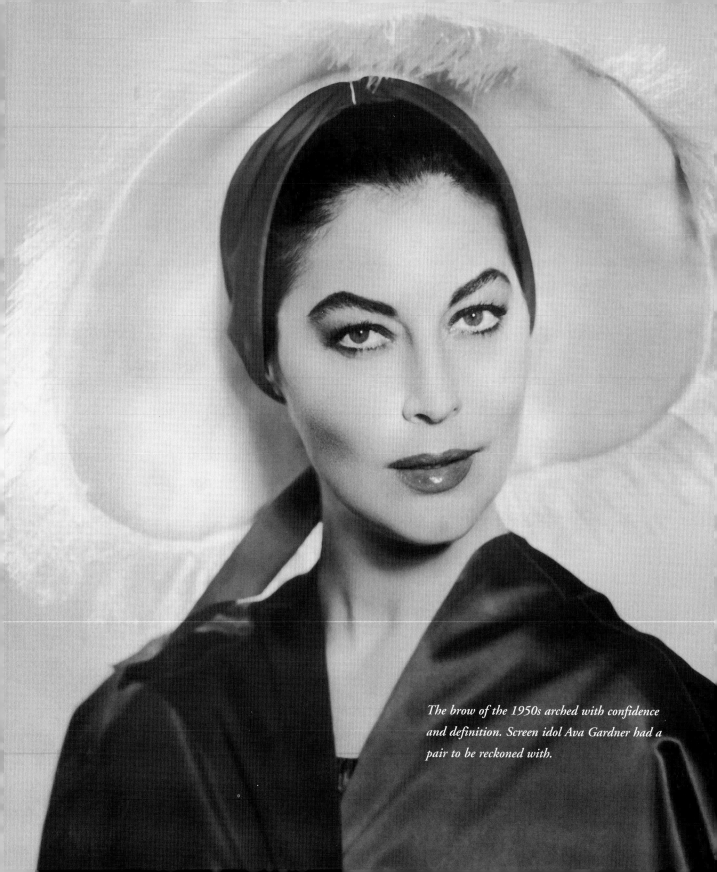

The brow of the 1950s arched with confidence and definition. Screen idol Ava Gardner had a pair to be reckoned with.

teenage heartbreaker, MGM's makeup department redid her look and established one of the single most memorable faces in film history.

Taylor's eyes, so lavender-blue they appear violet, were blessed with a double fringe of dark, luxuriant lashes. Her runaway brows, thick, black, and ready for shaping, were carved into the basic shape that she has maintained for forty years. Squared off nearest the nose, these are no escaping paisleys or frightened tadpoles. They march resolutely up to the top of the eye and take off into a sudden, downward angle, tapering off, long and low. These are major brows: wide, black, full, and expressive, as much a part of Taylor's personality as her violet eyes, her wasp waist, and her bounteous bosom.

As for the Hollywood blonde, she came along in the buxom, bawdy tradition of Jean Harlow and Mae West, with a few modern modifications. Her figure was defined by her breasts and her generous posterior, which, in 1950s fashion, were not shown off under slinky bias-cut satins, but in spangly, tight-as-paint, strapless evening gowns or abbreviated, two-piece white bathing suits. Marilyn Monroe, Mamie Van Doren, Jayne Mansfield, and Kim Novak were every mother's son's ultimate fantasy. Like their brunette sisters, the Va-Voom blondes all had something in common: black brows. Thick, manicured, and accented in dark pencil, these brows had to hold their own in an era where voluptuousness, coupled with juicy, slicked red lips, conferred an indelible image.

Of the four, Monroe has remained the most constant and memorable. She lived her life in Technicolor and was a perfectionist when it came to her image. While she was still Norma Jean Baker, an aspiring actress, she married a policeman named Jim Dougherty and then, after her transformation into a vulnerable screen goddess, she wed first the Yankee Clipper, Joe DiMaggio, then playwright Arthur Miller. She ran with the Sinatra Rat Pack and had rumored love affairs with both President John F. Kennedy and his brother, then-Attorney General Robert Kennedy. She was never out of the spotlight. She would spend hours getting her look into photographic shape, even making sure that every sequin on a sewn-on tight green dress was heading in the same direction, or that every hair was tousled to perfection.

Monroe's image, softened in later years by photographers Irving Penn and Bert Greene, was classic Bombshell. Her hair was peroxided into shades of golden, baby blond. Her face glowed, due in part to a fine layer of down that caught the light and made her appear to glow from within. Her makeup was very simple. It had to be. One misstep, and she would look hard and cheap. She wore iridescent shadow or a shimmer of gloss on her lids, lots of mascara, and lined only the top of her eyes, often fixing a few false lashes at the end of her top lid to give her eyes a sleepy, sexy squint. Her brows were neatly tweezed into the popular Diva Arch and darkened. It was not, however, the sophisticated, stylized brow of the fashion mannequin, but of the girl next door who happened to have a pneumatic body and a breathy little-girl voice. She was

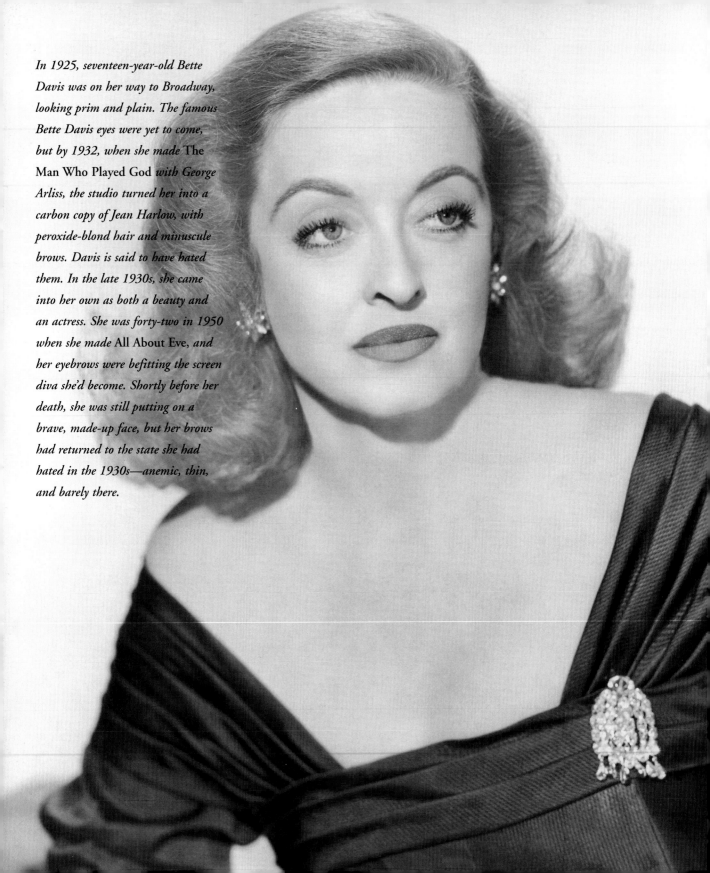

In 1925, seventeen-year-old Bette Davis was on her way to Broadway, looking prim and plain. The famous Bette Davis eyes were yet to come, but by 1932, when she made The Man Who Played God *with George Arliss, the studio turned her into a carbon copy of Jean Harlow, with peroxide-blond hair and minuscule brows. Davis is said to have hated them. In the late 1930s, she came into her own as both a beauty and an actress. She was forty-two in 1950 when she made* All About Eve, *and her eyebrows were befitting the screen diva she'd become. Shortly before her death, she was still putting on a brave, made-up face, but her brows had returned to the state she had hated in the 1930s—anemic, thin, and barely there.*

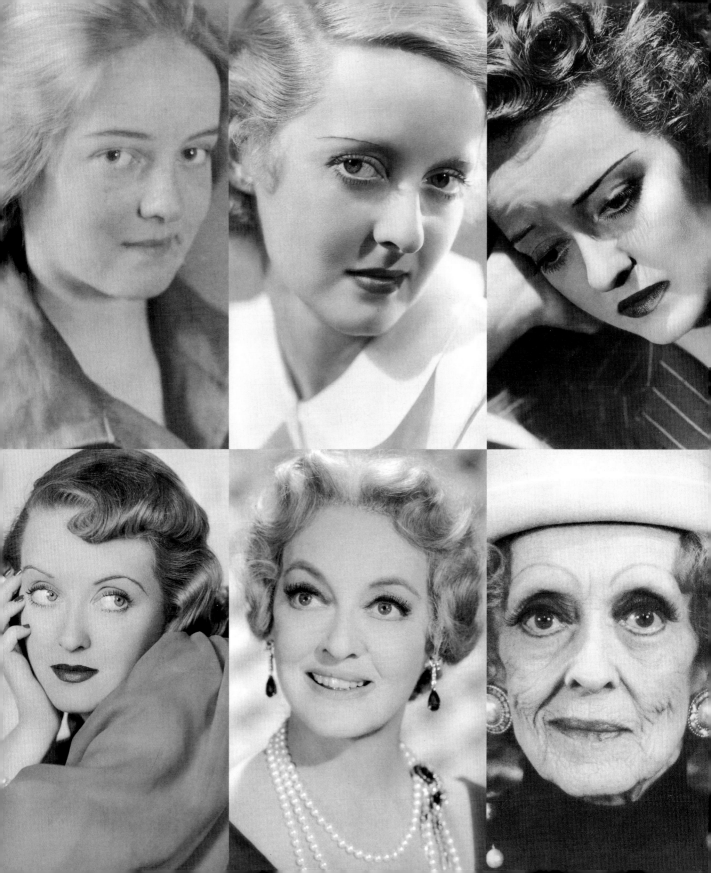

a natural beauty, but at the same time, there was something unnatural and otherworldly about her. Her hair was bright platinum, her lips as ruby as a maharajah's gem, and her brows fashionably dark and tweezed into perfection.

The Girls Next Door—Debbie Reynolds, Sandra Dee, Jane Powell, Doris Day, and Hope Lange—were pared down in comparison to the larger-than-life Siren or Bombshell. But they still exhibited the prevalent style of the day: a winged doe eye and a strong, dark brow, even on the blondes.

The other indelible look from the 1950s belonged to Audrey Hepburn, who came to represent the fresh-faced sprite, the Gamine, the enchantress, and yes, the Bohemian. Hepburn's makeup style was lifted directly from the ballet, which made sense. When she was a young girl in Holland and then in her teens in England, she had trained to be a ballerina. Her features fit the role: She had huge, direct, liquid brown eyes that could widen in amazement or express shyness or fear. Hepburn's eyebrows were shaped like an Asiatic prince's and drawn over her natural brows—thick, squared off, and set high above her eyes like graceful

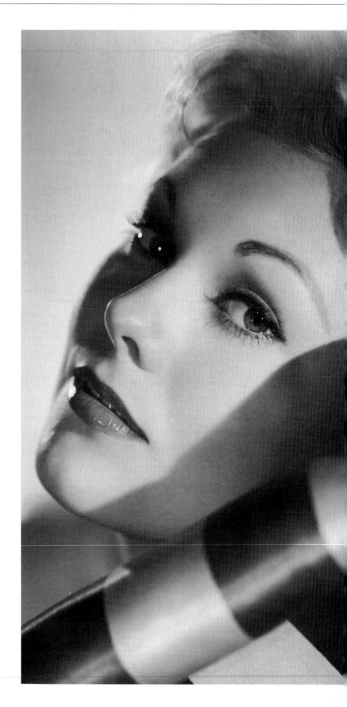

Another of Hollywood's 1950s Blond Bombshells, Kim Novak had artificially dark brows that contrasted with her fluffy blond hair. In reality, her own brows had been so overtweezed that they never grew back, and her makeup-assisted eyebrows were often done with a very careless, heavy hand.

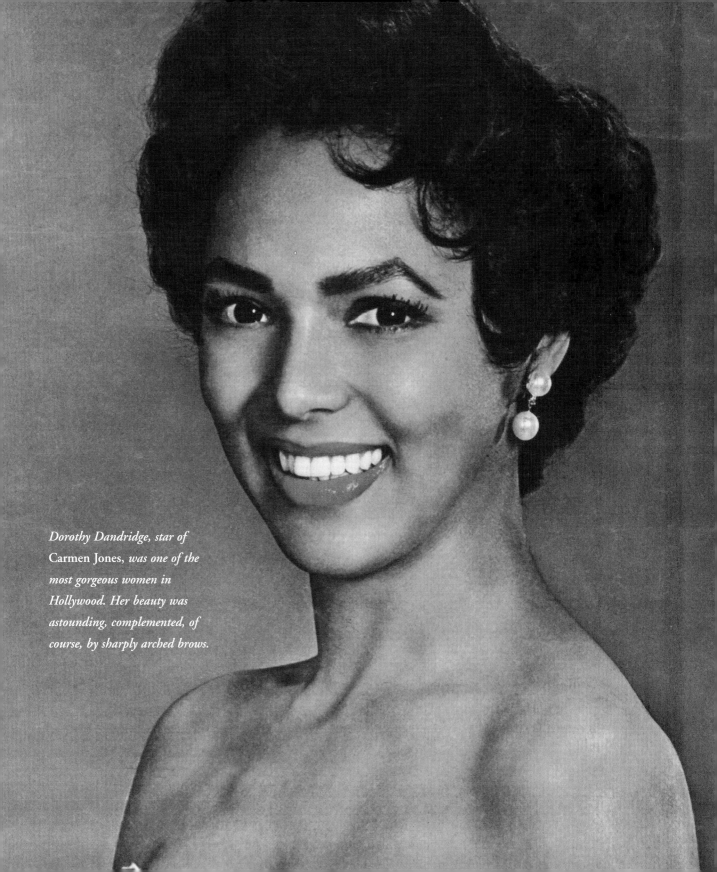

Dorothy Dandridge, star of **Carmen Jones,** *was one of the most gorgeous women in Hollywood. Her beauty was astounding, complemented, of course, by sharply arched brows.*

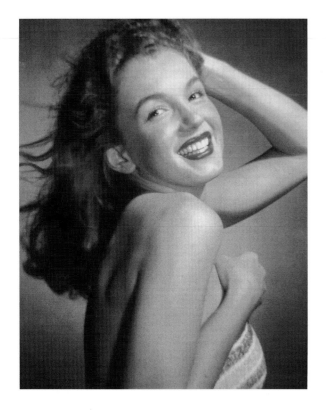

time, and when she and French couturier Hubert de Givenchy were paired off in *Sabrina*, it was a stylistic marriage made in heaven.

Toward the end of the decade, Hepburn appeared in *Funny Face,* which parodied the high-fashion model. Never had Hepburn looked quite so elegant. In a scene in a bohemian dive where her only costume was a black turtleneck sweater, slim Capri pants, and ballerina flats, she previewed the look that was to take over—the Beatnik, the Boho.

In the arty cafés of New York and the smoky *boîtes* of Paris, coffeehouse Circes like Juliette Greco—all long dark hair with bangs over raccoon eyes—modified the gentle, ladylike doe eye into the

feathers that tapered off with little or no arch. In the mid-Fifties, for films like *Roman Holiday* and *Sabrina,* and later onstage as the sea sprite who falls in love with a human in *Ondine*, Hepburn's eyebrows added to the air of birdlike girlishness and fragility that always sur-rounded her. In later years, for films like *Breakfast at Tiffany's* and *Charade*, her brows were lightened up into a more elegant arch.

Hepburn's hair was styled to emphasize her eyes, either pulled back into a ponytail with soft bangs or cut into a short pixie or gamin cut. Her lanky, boy-ish figure was perfect for the haute fashions of the

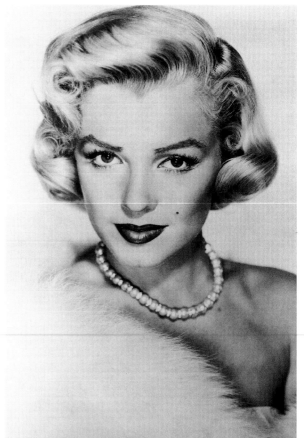

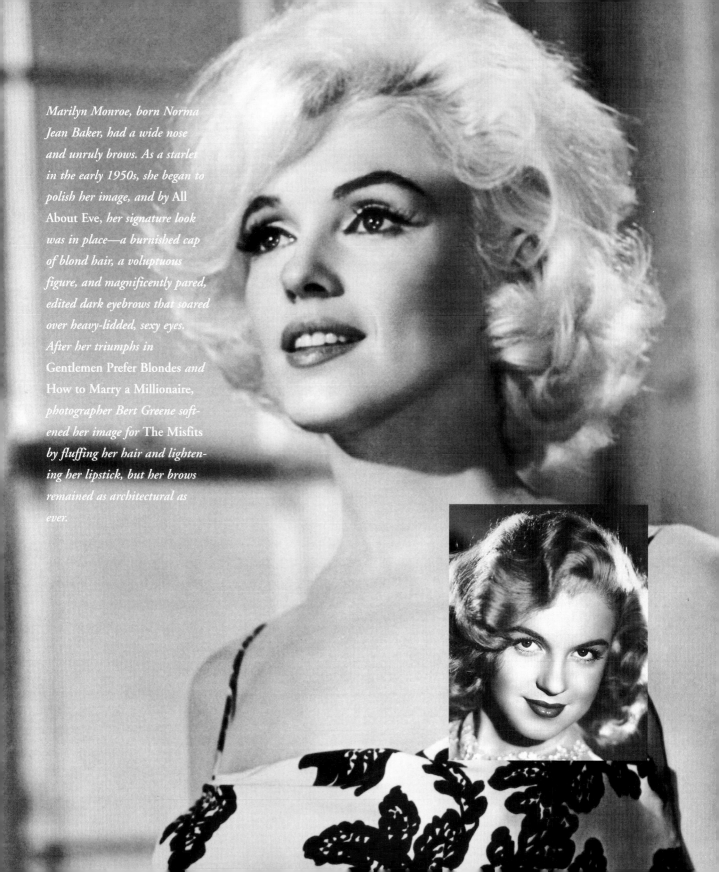

Marilyn Monroe, born Norma Jean Baker, had a wide nose and unruly brows. As a starlet in the early 1950s, she began to polish her image, and by All About Eve, *her signature look was in place—a burnished cap of blond hair, a voluptuous figure, and magnificently pared, edited dark eyebrows that soared over heavy-lidded, sexy eyes. After her triumphs in* Gentlemen Prefer Blondes *and* How to Marry a Millionaire, *photographer Bert Greene softened her image for* The Misfits *by fluffing her hair and lightening her lipstick, but her brows remained as architectural as ever.*

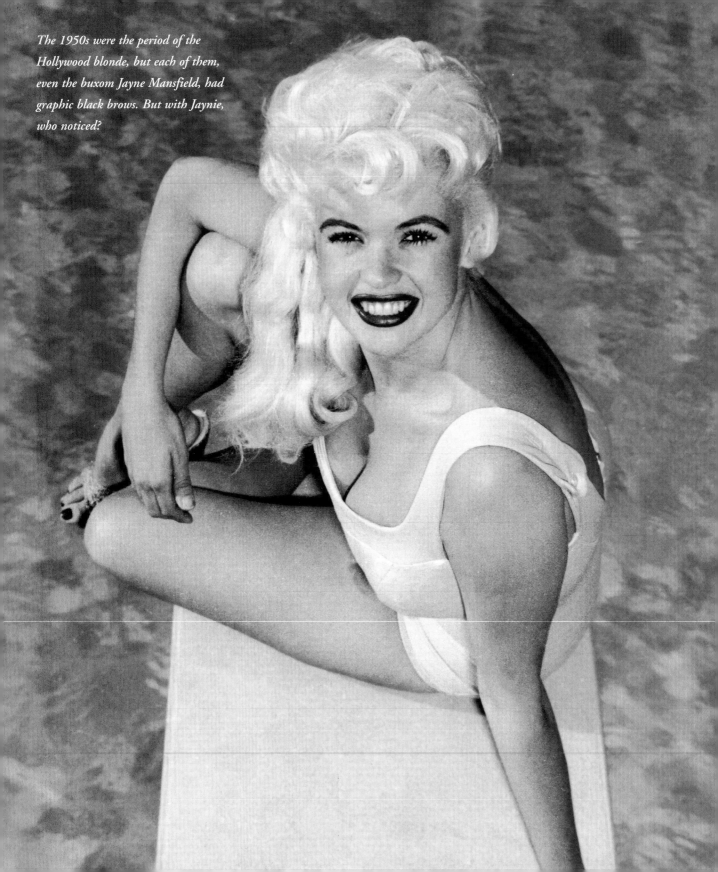

The 1950s were the period of the Hollywood blonde, but each of them, even the buxom Jayne Mansfield, had graphic black brows. But with Jaynie, who noticed?

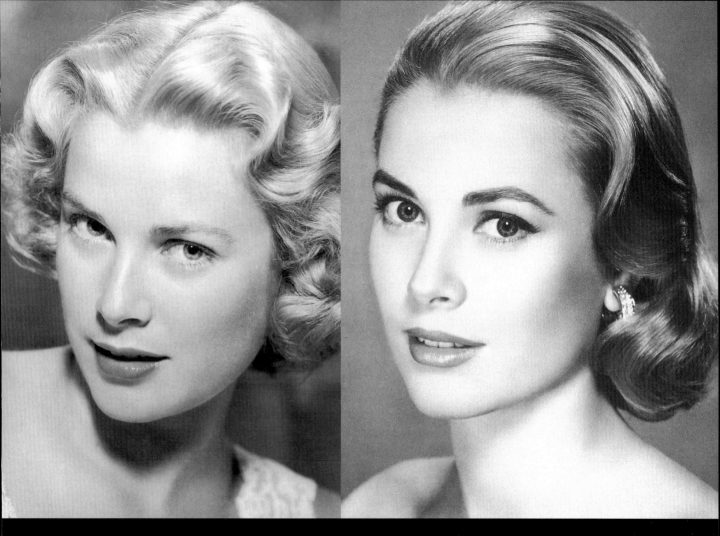

Grace Kelly, the former model and ice princess who married a real prince, was the iconic 1950s blonde. She was a natural beauty whom the studio makeup artists never ruined with too many cosmetics. They simply defined and emphasized her brows into an elegant arch. Kelly's fine bone structure and patrician carriage did the rest.

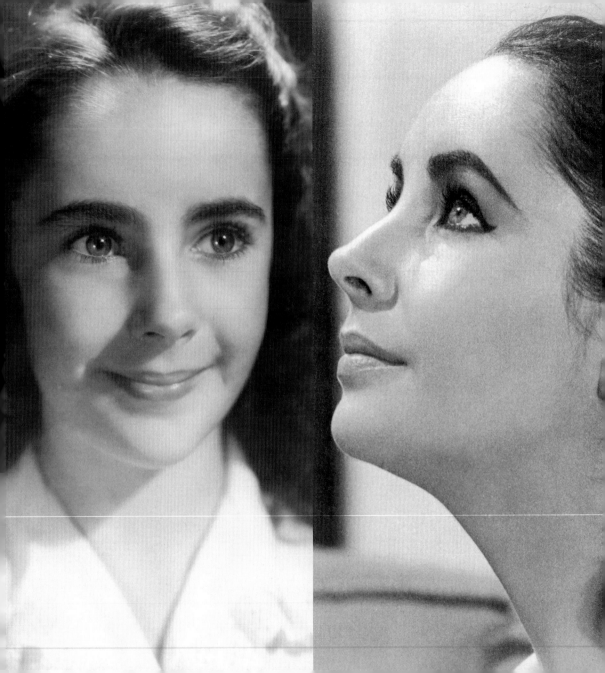

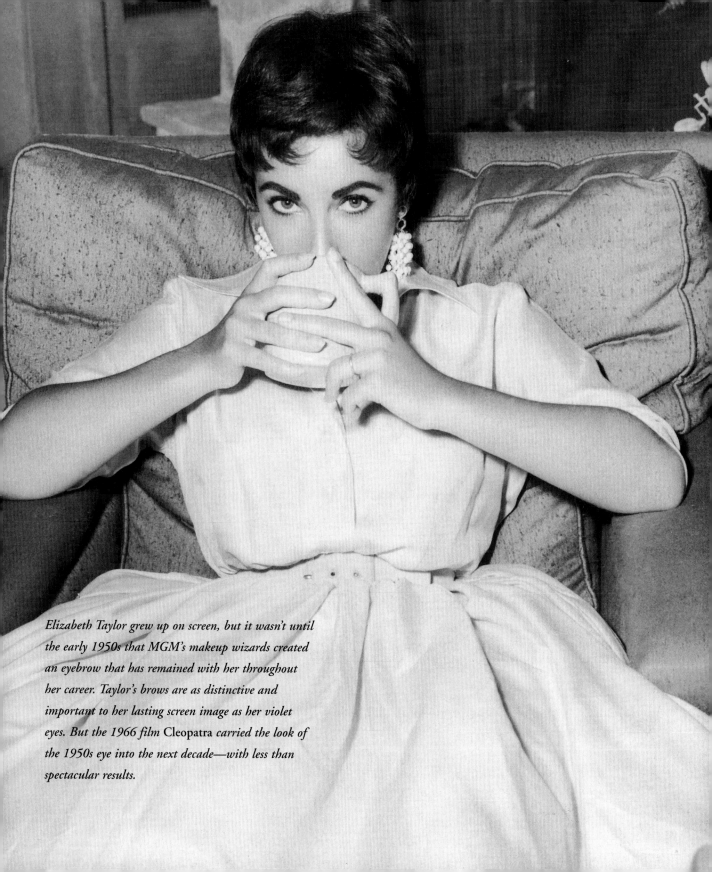

Elizabeth Taylor grew up on screen, but it wasn't until the early 1950s that MGM's makeup wizards created an eyebrow that has remained with her throughout her career. Taylor's brows are as distinctive and important to her lasting screen image as her violet eyes. But the 1966 film Cleopatra carried the look of the 1950s eye into the next decade—with less than spectacular results.

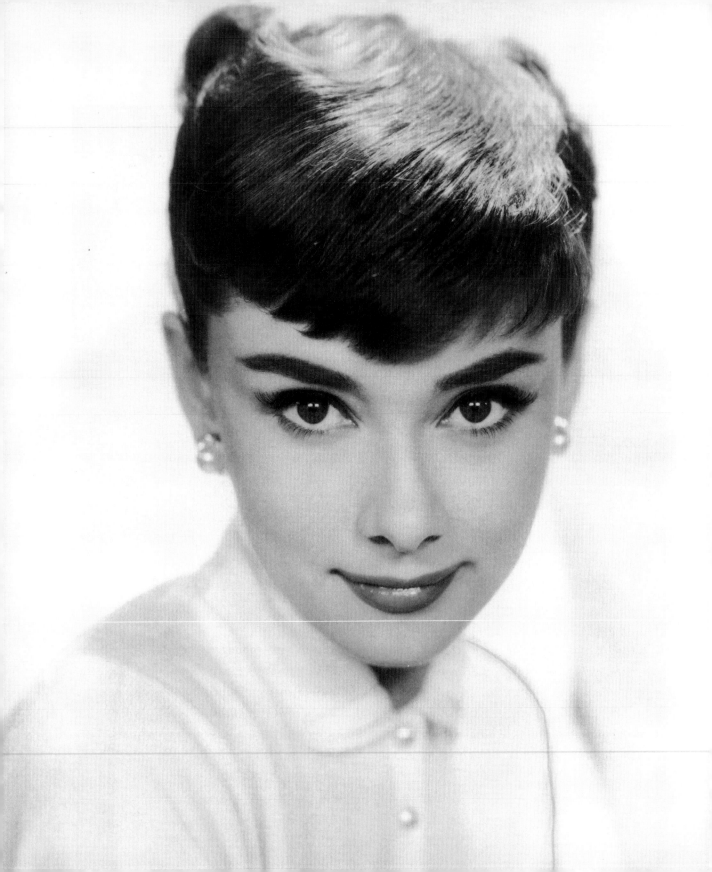

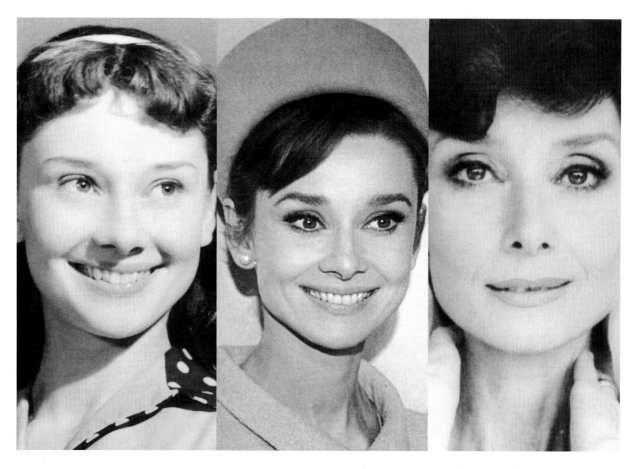

The quintessential 1950s eyebrow belonged to Audrey Hepburn, whose look was a translation of traditional ballet maquillage. Hepburn's brows were thickened with pencil drawn over and above her natural eyebrows in Roman Holiday *and* Sabrina. *Her doe-eyed innocence is one of the lasting images of the period. As she aged, her brows became lighter, shapelier, and, eventually, thinner.*

graphic Egyptian cat's eye by extending both upper and lower lines into a forceful ebony triangle at the outside corner. Lipstick was either nonexistent or lightened up with a thin coat of Max Factor's new concealer, Erase, underneath. And the eyebrow was as muscular as ever.

But change—coming via the avant garde stanzas of Allen Ginsberg's groundbreaking poetic rant, "Howl," or in the amphetamine-injected prose of Jack Kerouac's *On the Road*—was in the wind. With the advent of the Sixties, women and their faces would never be the same.

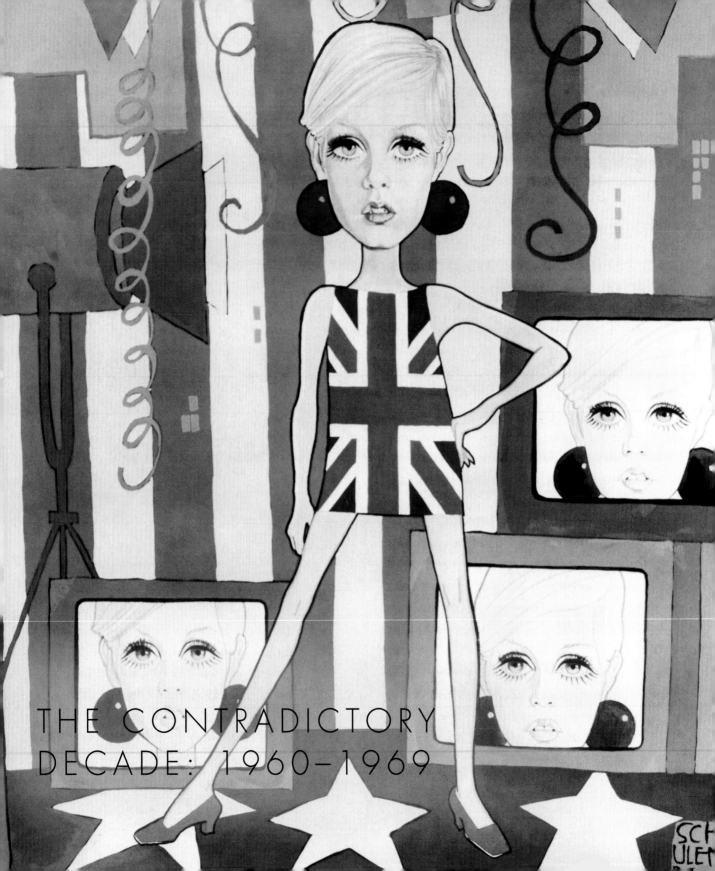

THE CONTRADICTORY
DECADE: 1960-1969

Perhaps no other decade divided in half stylistically as did the 1960s. Called the Soaring Sixties because of the Russian-American race into outer space, or the Swingin' Sixties because of the new freedoms granted women in the way they dressed, maquillaged, drank, drugged, made love, and partied, this was a decade of violent social change, one in which cosmetics played a diminishing role as the decade trundled on through the stridency of rock-and-roll and the morass of Vietnam.

With the election of the young, vital, and handsome John F. Kennedy to the White House in 1960, the decade began with hope in its heart. Kennedy's gracious, patrician wife, Jacqueline Bouvier Kennedy, was a camera-ready princess whose look was envied and copied. She wore simple clothes—Sabrina-necked, sleeveless skimmer dresses with matching coats and pert little pillbox hats perched atop her brunette bouffant.

Jackie, as Americans loved to call her, had strong features that needed enhancement, not camouflage. Her makeup was ladylike: light pink/coral lipsticks; very little eyeshadow; eyes lined in the 1950s manner with a neat, winged black line; just enough mascara to dress, not emphasize, her lashes; and thick, natural

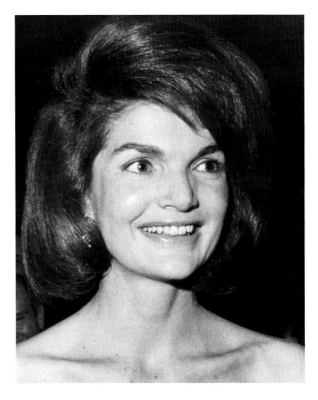

Early in the 1960s, when Jacqueline Bouvier Kennedy ruled Washington as first lady, she developed her own simply tailored look with the help of couturier Oleg Cassini, but she retained the 1950s ideal of beauty with coral lipstick and strong, carefully arched, and exquisitely groomed brows.

Twiggy epitomized Swingin' London with her short, gamine hair, her glistening pink lips, and her round, innocent eyes made even more dramatic with painted-on lashes. Her eyebrows, however, were skinny, flyaway affairs, almost an afterthought to her dramatic eye treatment.

brows that slanted upward with a slightly exotic cast that were brushed and tweezed free of excess hair.

When her husband was killed by an assassin's bullet on November 22, 1963, the 1950s were officially over. Where coeds were once wearing box-pleated skirts, cashmere twin sets, good pearls, and Spalding saddle shoes with Adler sweat socks to class,

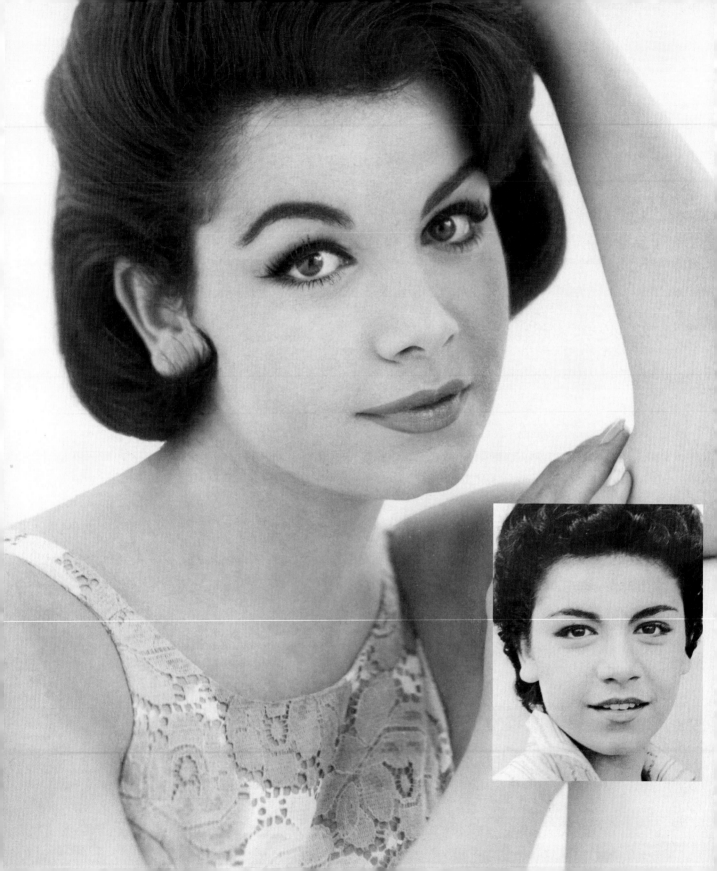

they now affected Levi's, Frye boots, and green Harvard bookbags. Rent strikes and other campus-originated protests were changing the face of young America, accompanied by the clarion call of rock-and-roll.

Elvis Presley was out of the Army and into movies, and the Beach Boys were crooning their California surfin' music and extolling the pleasures of the California blonde—a willowy, long-haired girl with long, sun-tanned legs and eyebrows bleached by the summer sun.

But the British were coming, bringing with them the subversive sensibilities of four mop-topped boys—John, Paul, George, and Ringo—and a whole mess of fashion-forward outrageousness. The Beatles' London Look came straight from the boutiques of Biba and Mary Quant. Both designers catered to the Mod girl in her abbreviated miniskirt and poor boy sweater (fashion inventions that put Quant on the map) or to the romantic Chelsea girl in her velvet Edwardian suits, flowing satin skirts, lacy jabots, and long, flowing hair.

In Quant's Chelsea boutique, you could buy her clothes and makeup, which was packaged in rounded black containers with her stylized four-leaf-clover logo on top. Quant touted a naked face and well-dressed eyes. "Lipstick," she advised in her book

As a Walt Disney Mouseketeer, Annette Funicello was blessed with dark, thick brows that only got darker and thicker as her career progressed into beach party movies.

Quant on Quant, "is kept to a pale gloss and the only area where you can go to town is around the eyes. There, you can use a lot of eyeshadow, eyeliner, and lots of mascara, plus false eyelashes, even false eyebrows, I should think, provided you've managed to master the art of putting them on and keeping them in place." (There is no record as to whether people actually did use false brows like the Restoration beauties who terrorized the mouse population of London for their hides.)

The message from London was, anything goes. Just as long as it was creative. It was the cult of the individual beauty, female role models who were not members of the cookie-cutter set from the previous decade. In the early 1960s, oddball beauties such as the six-foot-four-inch-tall, androgynous Prussian countess-turned-fashion model Verushka (born Vera Gottlieb von Lehndorff) and chanteuse Barbra Streisand gloried in their offbeat looks by emphasizing their best features. In Streisand's case, it was her delicious sloe eyes, which she painted like Cleopatra. Verushka was often photographed in the nude, painted up like a python or a panther to show off her lean, muscular body. She was muse to designer Giorgio Sant'Angelo, who dressed her in fringes and Rich Hippie leathers and advocated the use of fingers instead of pencils to soften and smudge makeups. "Eyebrows," he declared in 1961 in French *Vogue*, "should be fixed with false eyelash glue applied with a toothbrush. Brows may be brushed straight up to produce an ethereal, feline beauty."

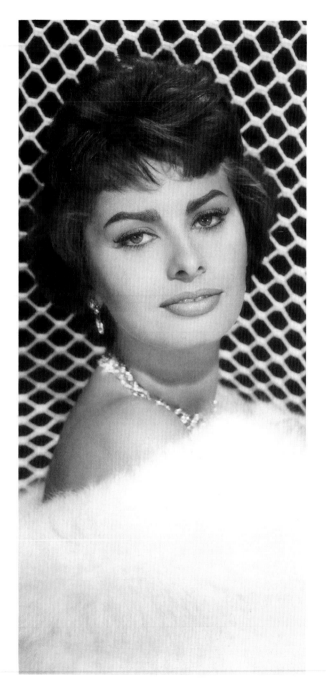

London sent two vastly different models to America: Jean Shrimpton, whose classic romantic aura spawned a fashion look that lasted the entire decade, and the waiflike, fifteen-year-old Lesley Hornby, a.k.a. Twiggy, whose spindly legs and gawky coltish sassiness were in complete contradiction to all the standards of *haute-couture* beauty that had preceded her in the elegant Fifties. Jean, called "The Shrimp," was the model you used if you wanted a soft, decadent Edwardian look. She wore velvet coats and frilled blouses like a female fop; her brows were thick and groomed and her eyes were soft. The perfect symmetry of her features made her stunning.

Twiggy was the invention of a hairdresser and model manager who called himself Justin Villeneuve. As small and downright skinny as she was, she presented the perfect physique for the fashions of the day as well as the fantasy makeups coming from the paint pots of makeup artists like Elizabeth Arden's Pablo Manzoni, who would decorate an eye like a Christmas tree. Often he would obscure half of Twiggy's face with a baroquely painted eye—a plume of peacock color culminating in a feather-decorated brow; a glittery

Italy's gift to American filmdom is Sophia Loren, whose earthy sensuality glowed from the screen. In the 1950s, her brows were heavy and defined. In the 1960s, however, she started a trend. She shaved her brows off and repenciled them with teeny, individual strokes, but many Youth Quakers learned the hard way that sometimes brows don't grow back.

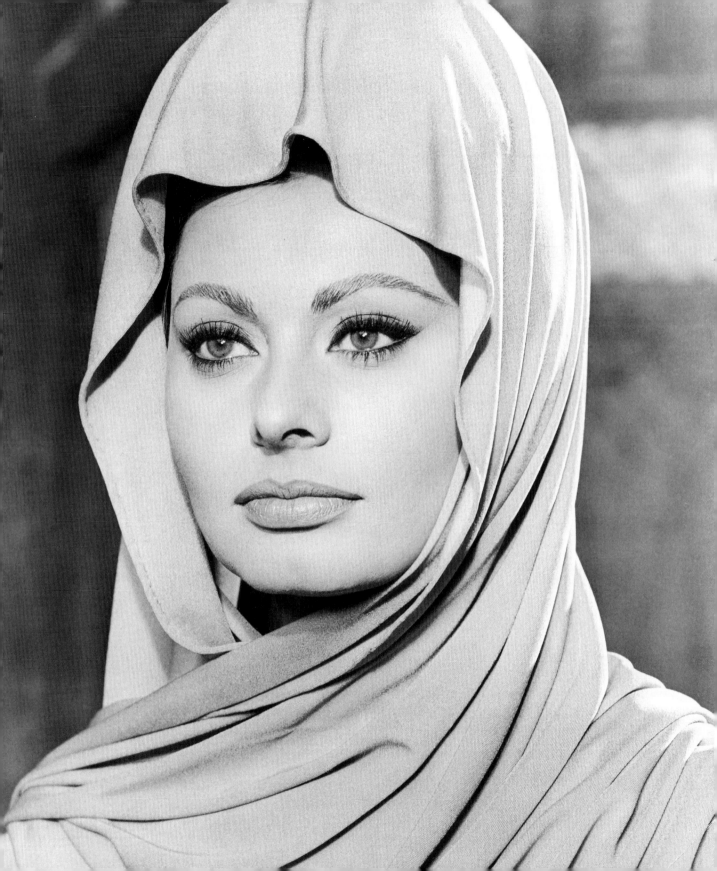

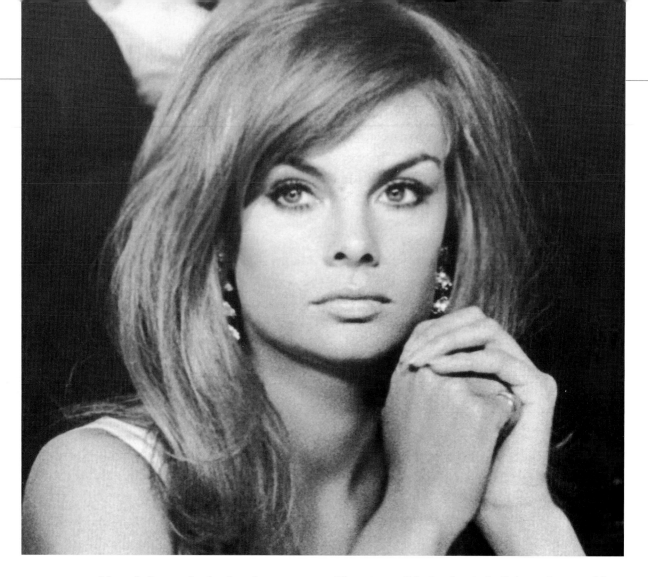

snow scene with real diamonds glued to her sparse arches; or glitter paving the surface of her lids from lashline to brow arch. Anything went. Flowers, birds, feathers, and later on, the Day-Glo psychedelia of madly scribbled paisleys and Op-Art patterns.

Young designers coming out of London and Paris were riffing on the same theme: the Youth Quake. While Mary Quant was trend-setting in London, in Paris, André Courrèges with his architec-

The epitome of the London Look Chelsea girl was model Jean Shrimpton, a.k.a. The Shrimp, whose expressive brows still echoed the 1950s.

tural, welt-seamed white miniskirts worn with black, ribbed turtlenecks, black tights, and white go-go boots vied with Paco Rabanne, who made modern chain mail clothing out of geometric plastic discs held together with tiny metal jump rings. The con-

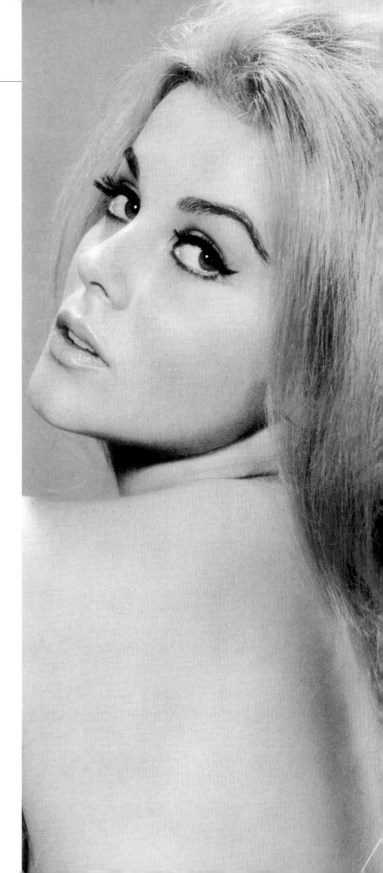

temporary French girl who wore these space-agey creations called herself the Yé-Yé Girl, named after the adorable pack of groupies who ran after rocker Johnny Halliday. While Rabanne and Courrèges catered to a younger, hipper crowd, Parisian *haute couture* was kept alive by Pierre Cardin, who made major changes to men's clothing construction. He got guys out of their stodgy, boxy, baggy Brooks Brothers suits and into clothes with nipped-in waists, daring plaids, and pleated trousers.

Courrèges wanted to sweep away all vestiges of the recent past by erasing the image of the 1950s screen siren with her red lacquered nails, red lips, and heavy brows. On the runway, he used an entire United Nations of models—Asian and black women, redheads, and gamines like Twiggy. He stuffed his models' hair under Day-Glo Dynel wigs, which contrasted hugely with his all-white palette and dictated strong eye makeup to support the look. Models used thick, black eyeliner on both upper and lower lashlines, separated by a small parallel line of white between to open the eyes. The eyebrow was an afterthought, sometimes obliterated with makeup and redrawn so it wouldn't conflict with the eye.

In the States, the modern girl came out of the Warhol studio in the personage of Edie Sedgwick.

When she burst on the scene as a Chicago teenager in Bye-Bye Birdie, *redheaded Ann-Margret grew into an actress and dynamic nightclub performer whose eyebrows were tweezed and defined into a catlike arch.*

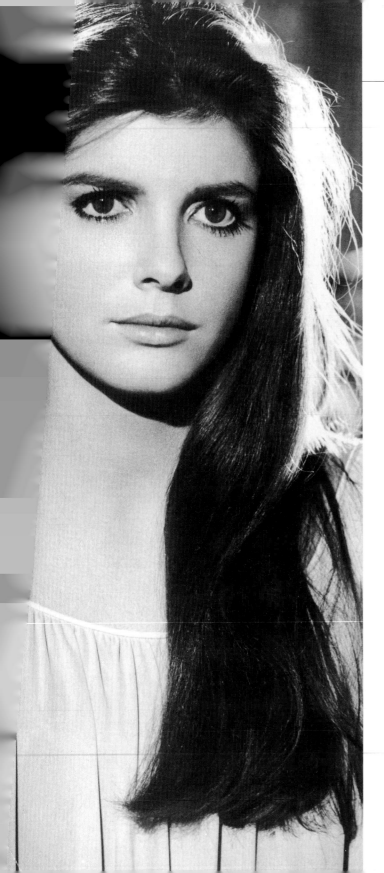

Silver was her color (as were the walls of Warhol's Chelsea studio in New York). A tragic character who died from amphetamine poisoning, Edie was nonetheless a strikingly adorable girl, as waifish as Twiggy and much more wellborn. (Warhol had a penchant for attracting disaffected rich girls who wanted some thrills in their lives.) Like Twiggy, Edie had a chameleonesque quality to her. She painted her face with silver patterns, wore light pink lipstick, and tweezed her brows down to tiny arcs.

In fact, in the earlier part of the decade, the eyebrow became considerably smaller and less prominent. If the 1950s were the Eyebrow Decade of the century, the 1960s were all about hair and eyes. Never was this more true than with tawny-maned Brigitte Bardot, the French sex kitten who made cinema history when she appeared in the buff in *And God Created Woman*. The protégée of director Roger Vadim (later married to Jane Fonda in her *Barbarella* days), Bardot was a voluptuous beauty.

Anomalies in the midst of all this rock-and-roll frenzy were Elizabeth Taylor and the monumentally expensive Columbia Pictures production of *Cleopatra*, which was released in 1966. Despite the scandal that surrounded the film—Taylor left her husband, singer

In the early 1960s, fueled by the Beach Boys' paeans to surfin' and California girls, the nation fell in love with a pair of golden girls, Katharine Ross and Candice Bergen, whose makeup was pared down and whose brows were allowed to flourish naturally.

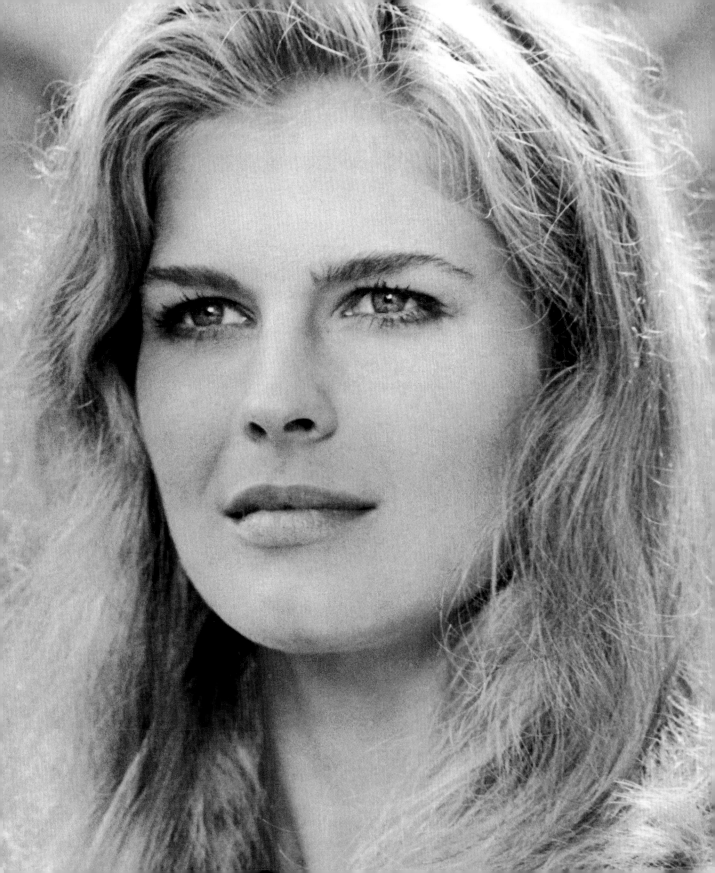

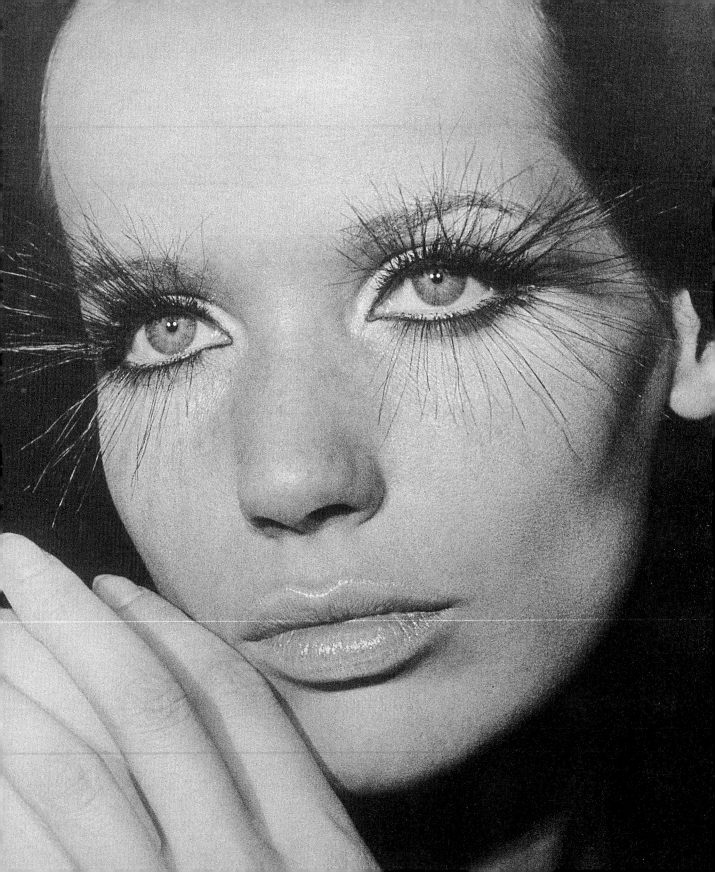

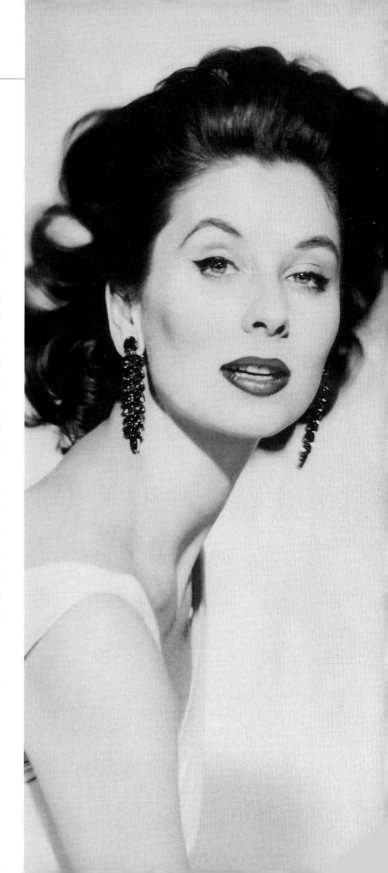

With her tall, athletic body, Prussian-born Countess Verushka was the couture photographers' darling because there wasn't a hairpiece or pot of body paint she didn't like. In the mid-Sixties, the era of the eyebrows was definitely over. Eyes in; eyebrows out.

Eddie Fisher, for Richard Burton, who was inconveniently married at the time—the film was an expensive white elephant. And her elaborate Cleo eyes, with their turquoise blue and green lids and fantastic black liner, were not a style-setting success. Taylor looked like Taylor, only more so, with her heavy eyebrows made even darker and oppressive by massive applications of black pencil. If there was an anticipated fad, it never materialized, for when the film hit, the decade was about to take a radical change that would eliminate the desire for and the obvious use of cosmetics.

As the Sixties went on, well groomed wasn't an adjective any mother would use to refer to her daughter. As Bob Dylan sang, "The Times, They Are A-Changin'." The Vietnam War gained in intensity, and more and more American boys were plucked out of jobs and college and sent into the steamy jungles of Southeast Asia to fight the Viet Cong. Students hit the streets in protest. The years after 1965 were a tumult of causes, marches, sit-ins, protests, and social change. Female students started

Suzy Parker made the transition from modeling to films. Her arrogant brows cemented her look.

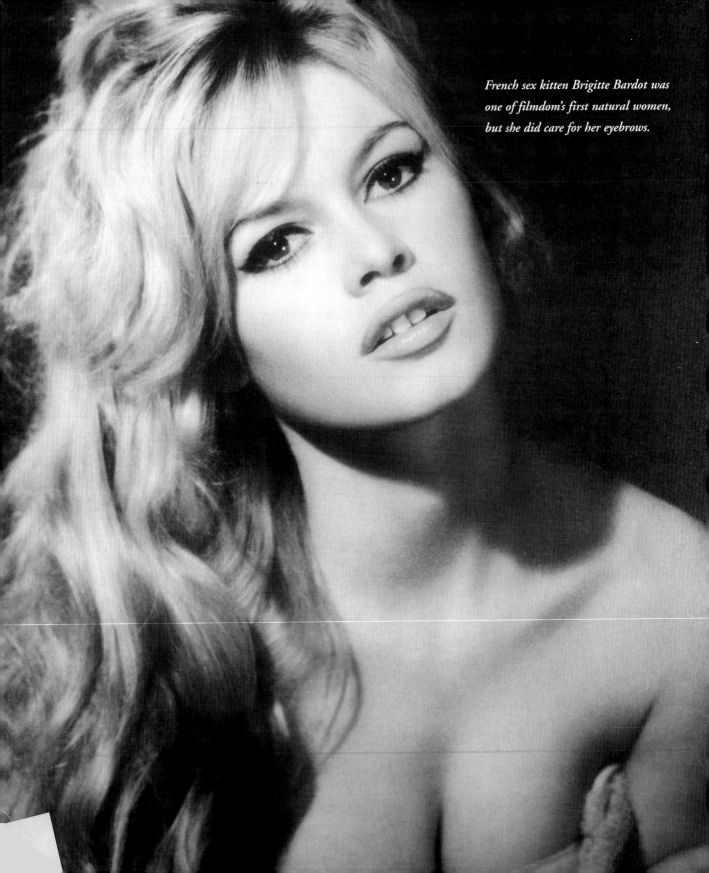

French sex kitten Brigitte Bardot was one of filmdom's first natural women, but she did care for her eyebrows.

looking like carbon copies of their boyfriends. They let their hair grow long and straight (and if it curled, they painstakingly ironed it or set it on orange juice cans all night to flatten it), and donned flannel shirts, blue jeans, Frye boots, and fatigue jackets. The latter half of the 1960s was not a particularly elegant era for the eyebrow. Young women, if they didn't do without makeup altogether, were happy to splash on pungent patchouli oil, stick flowers in their hair, and let their eyebrows go where they wanted to.

Dubbed "hippies" by antiwar activist Jerry Rubin, America's college-aged youth hit the road.

French film beauty Catherine Deneuve was Europe's answer to the Golden Girl. Her hair was long and blond, her clothes were by Yves Saint Laurent, and her couture eyebrows, neither too thick nor too thin, arched with elegant symmetry.

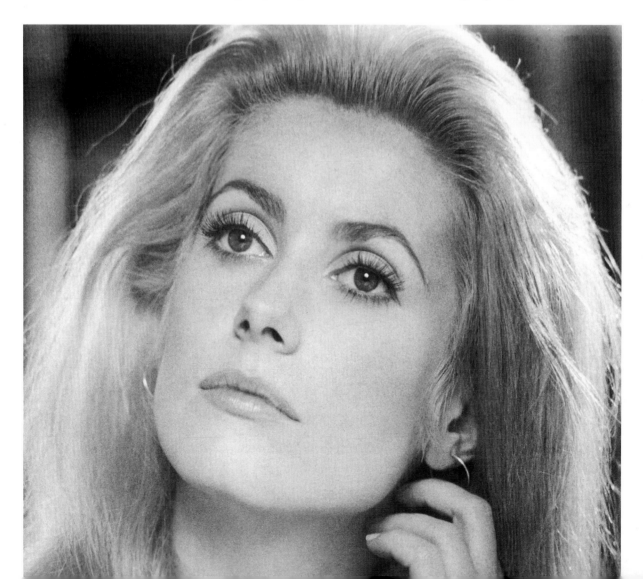

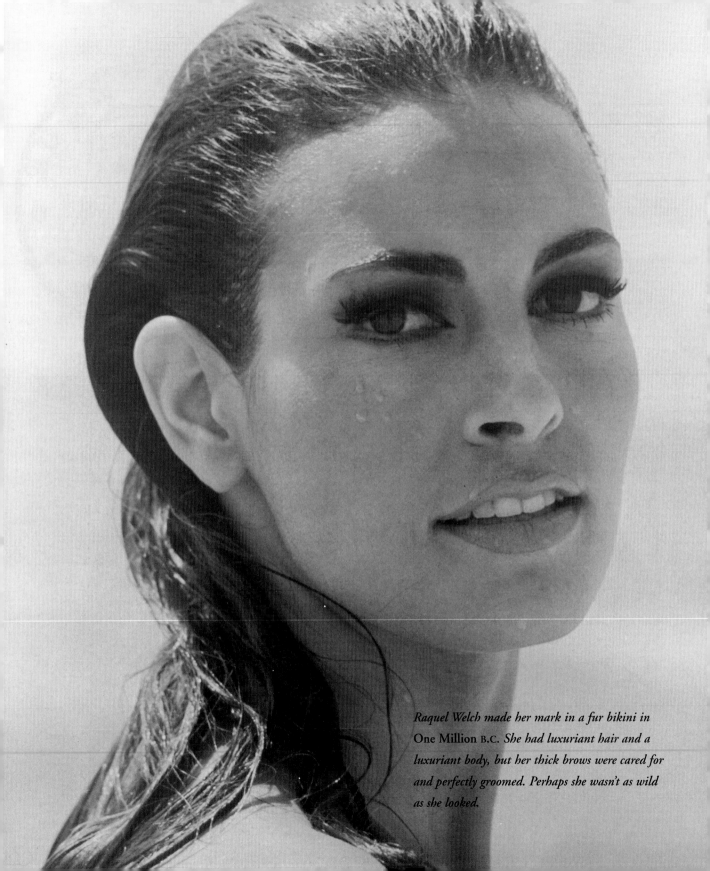

Raquel Welch made her mark in a fur bikini in One Million B.C. *She had luxuriant hair and a luxuriant body, but her thick brows were cared for and perfectly groomed. Perhaps she wasn't as wild as she looked.*

Former model and fashion stylist Ali MacGraw had dark hair and such overpowering brows that they needed constant attention, especially in films such as Goodbye, Columbus *and* Love Story. *Her contradictory screen image was a cross between sultry exoticism, the All-American Girl, and the hippie Bohemian.*

Some came to crash pads in San Francisco's Haight-Ashbury, kicked back, smoked marijuana, tripped on LSD, and followed bands like the Grateful Dead and the Jefferson Airplane. Others went back to the land, living in communal farms in Big Sur; Woodstock, New York; Eugene, Oregon; Taos, New Mexico; or in the Santa Cruz Mountains. They dabbled in Eastern mysticism, took drugs that made them hallucinate, revered Native American Indian customs, and translated what they had dreamed or learned into the back-to-nature, ethnically flavored Flower Child fashion.

New York's clothing designers, whose influence was almost derailed by the middle of the decade, copied the hippie style and created a hybrid fashion of beads, fringes, Palomino-colored suedes, and Hopi turquoise called the Rich Hippie, seen on actress/models Candice Bergen and Ali MacGraw and songstresses like Joni Mitchell, Judy Collins, and the Mamas and the Papas' Michelle Phillips, none of whom used all that many cosmetics. If it wasn't for Ali MacGraw's naturally thick brows, which she kept under control with a brush and judiciously spare tweezing, the eyebrow would have been an afterthought.

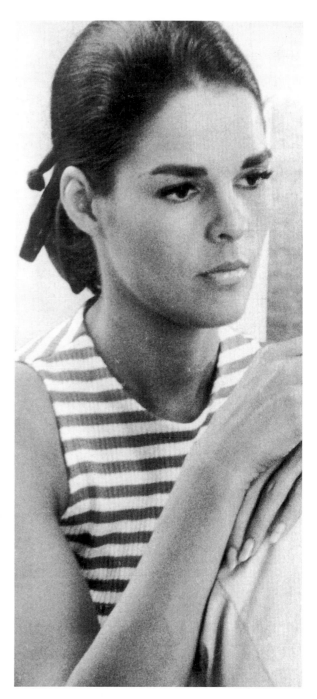

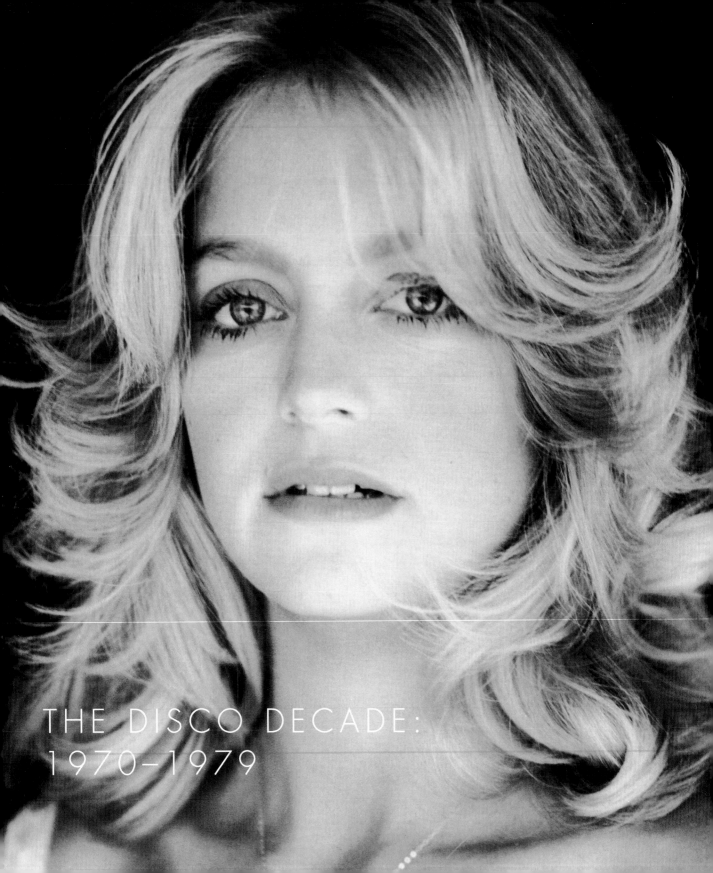

THE DISCO DECADE:
1970–1979

Were it not for bad taste, the 1970s would have had no taste at all. This is the decade that almost killed couture. With all the manmade fabrics floating around, one wondered, "How many polyesters died for *that* shirt?" This was the decade of the hip-rider bell-bottom, the platform shoe, and Farrah Fawcett's leonine mane of double-tiered feathery waves.

Despite the proletarian taste levels and the "let's party" attitude, this was the decade where women made serious inroads into the male status quo. The women's movement, championed by Germaine Greer, Gloria Steinem, and Betty Friedan, produced serious sociological change: Women became more sexual, more obvious. If the 1960s was a druggy decade in which unmarried girls and boys lived together, the 1970s belonged to the aggressive female who thought very little of asking a guy out or even sleeping with him after a first date, often never to see him again. Pleasure-bent, women were attempting to learn the no-guilt attitudes that men had held for years. They danced all night in smoke-filled discotheques, slugging back tequila shooters and snorting cocaine.

The new sexuality translated into provocative

Goldie Hawn, who made her show biz splash as a body-painted, bikini-clad pixie on NBC's outrageous variety show Rowan and Martin's Laugh-In, *never lost her sparkle or her signature look: tousled, multi-blonded hair, and long bangs that always obscure her dark taupe brows.*

clothes. When women burned their bras in protest during the early years of the women's movement, many young women simply took them off and went braless under sheer silk or lace blouses. They wore halters cut down to the waist in the back and hip-rider jeans with elephant bell-bottoms that at their extreme grew as wide as forty inches.

In the Disco Era, the face was all about glitter. Madeleine Mono's Arabian Light disco shadows were vivid powders flecked with mica that went on the lid wet or dry. They picked up the flash of the strobe or the gleaming shards of light sent around a club when a spotlight hit a mirrored ball. Lips were fairly neutral and often painted with brownish lipstick. And eyebrows were reduced to skinny commas, paisleys, or tadpoles—shortened, narrowed, and pared to feathery diacritical marks above the eye.

There was a certain stylistic schizophrenia to the Seventies. As couture was fighting for its life in Paris against the rising trend of unnatural fabrics and cheaply made, garishly patterned hot pants ensembles, couturier Yves Saint Laurent was sending models down the runway in the haughty makeups of the 1950s—the incredibly arched brow over red lips. A strong face above equally strong, masculine clothes. In Paris the 1970s brought Le Smoking, the trouser-suit tuxedo that has become one of YSL's signature looks, and the khaki safari jacket, which was adapted and co-opted in the 1980s by Ralph Lauren.

Contrast YSL's elegant twist on androgyny with the Disco Queen in her hip riders and cropped top,

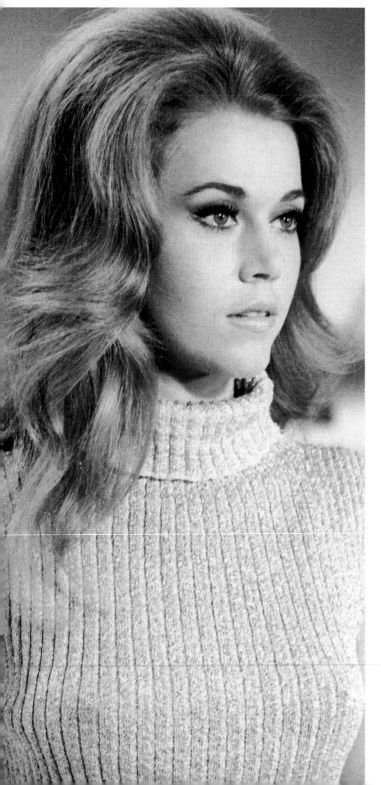

often covered in metallic paillettes as big as quarters, with eyes doused in mica shadows so flashy that you needed sunglasses at night. The men were equally as outrageous. Glam rockers like David Bowie as Ziggy Stardust, Elton John, and T. Rex's Marc Bolan tweaked the gender line with scandalous characters whose costumes were fantasies of lamé, velvet, campy Ming the Merciless shoulders, and thigh-high boots. Their faces were covered in strange Kabuki makeups. As the space alien Ziggy, Bowie, a former art student whose image changed from album to album, shaved off his eyebrows, as did his wife, Angie.

Later on in the decade, the high-fashion model ended her hippie phase. Not the scrawny androgyne that Twiggy, Peggy Moffitt, or Penelope Tree had been, this was a new crop of girly-girls. Rosie Vela, Rene Russo, and Patti Hanson were athletic-looking women with long tresses, golden complexions, and naturally thick brows. Their faces were polished and contoured. Deep brown-burgundy blush filled out the hollows under their cheekbones, which had been brushed with highlighter for an edgy gleam. They wore triple-tiered eye shadow—a neutral beige near the lashline, dark brown in the crease, and paper white under the brow. There were few false lashes.

When Roger Vadim got hold of the young Jane Fonda and turned her into one of his patented sex kittens in Barbarella, *he remade her by pouffing out her hair with fake pieces and defining her eyebrows. She took on a more serious attitude in the Seventies in* Klute *and* The China Syndrome, *and her brows got slightly thinner.*

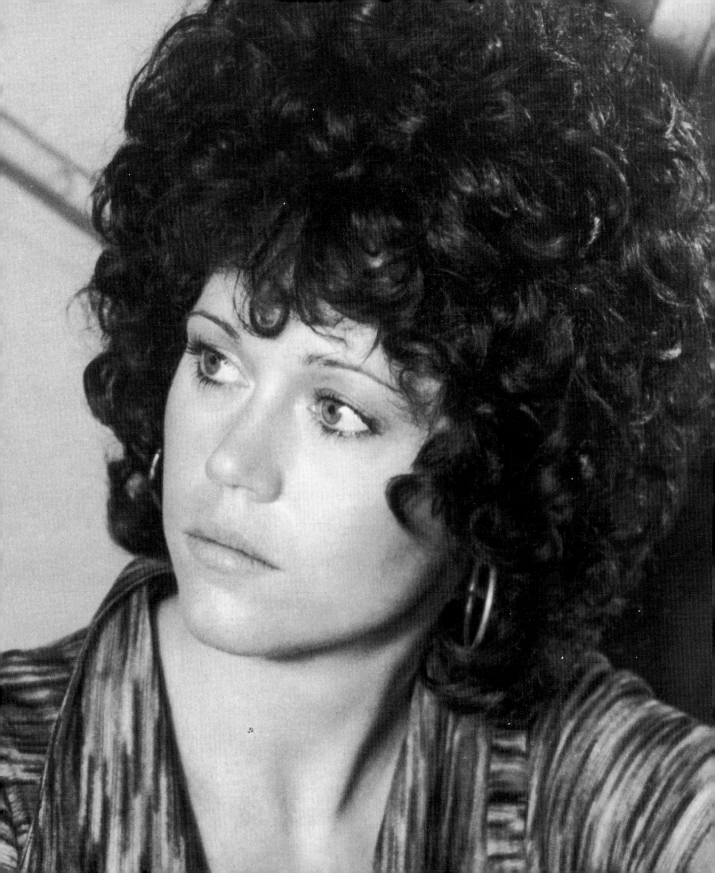

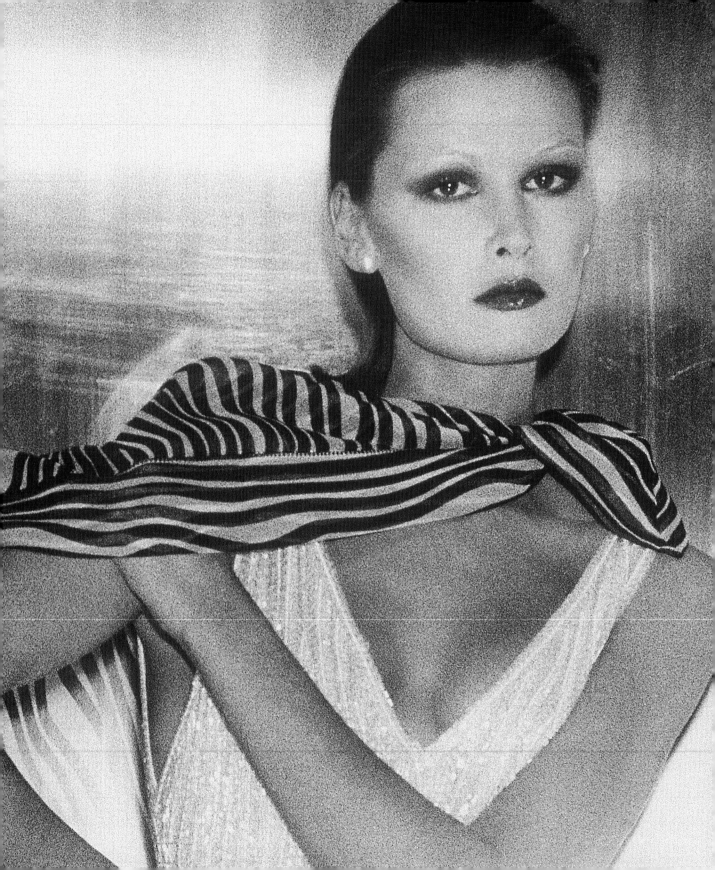

For emphasis, eyes were circled all around with a teensy, precise black line. There was nothing minimalist about the look, except the brows, which had been tweezed nearly as thin as the brow was in the 1930s. The prevailing style was a rounded contour pared of excess hair. Only a few sparse filaments supported the arch.

Things were soon to change. There was a movement in London that would impact American fashion for years. The Punks were coming. The Sex Pistols arrived in the States in 1977. They were rude, crude, and boisterous, and their following had an F— You attitude that had not been seen since Gertie bobbed her hair. With their quasi-S&M sensibility—heavy Doc Marten lace-up, steel-toed boots; fetish leathers; chrome-studded dog collars; and their shaven-sided, Day-Glo–dyed, spiked Mohawks—they were as shocking to look at as to listen to. The girls wore overtly pale faces like those of vampires and rimmed their eyes with kohl, often into masklike raccoon pools, painted their nails black, and wore black lipstick. Eyebrows (and just about any other facial feature—ears, noses, tongues) were modified—shaved off altogether or pierced with an assortment of safety pins, silver studs, delicate rings, spikes, and miniature barbells.

The look was designed to horrify parents and to warn the squares to stay out of their way. Unlike the hippie Flower Children, whose style was basically ethnic and soft-looking, the Punkers were aggressive in

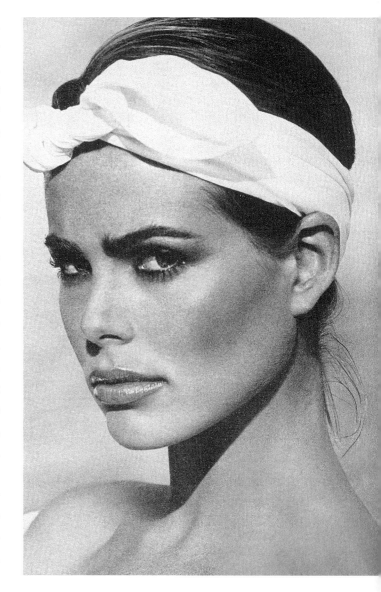

During the Seventies, a decade of bad taste and fashion contradiction, the eyebrow came in and out of prominence, alternately shaved off altogether or allowed to grow in width and intensity.

117

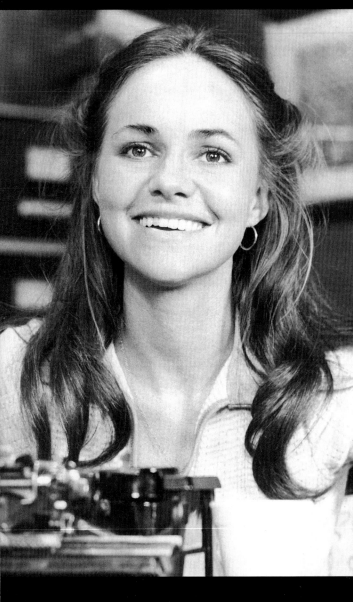

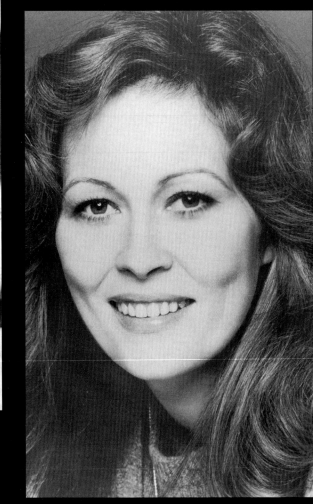

The epitome of elegance in films like Chinatown, The Eyes of Laura Mars, *and the original* Thomas Crown Affair, *model-turned-film-diva Faye Dunaway has played up her classic bone structure with neutral makeups and very little variation on her face. Only her eyebrows have fallen prey to trends: In the Seventies they were tweezed down for* Chinatown, *and they stayed that thin for years.*

In the Seventies, when Sally Field made Norma Rae, *her flying paisley brows, with big, rounded heads that tapered off into narrow tails, were typical of the period.*

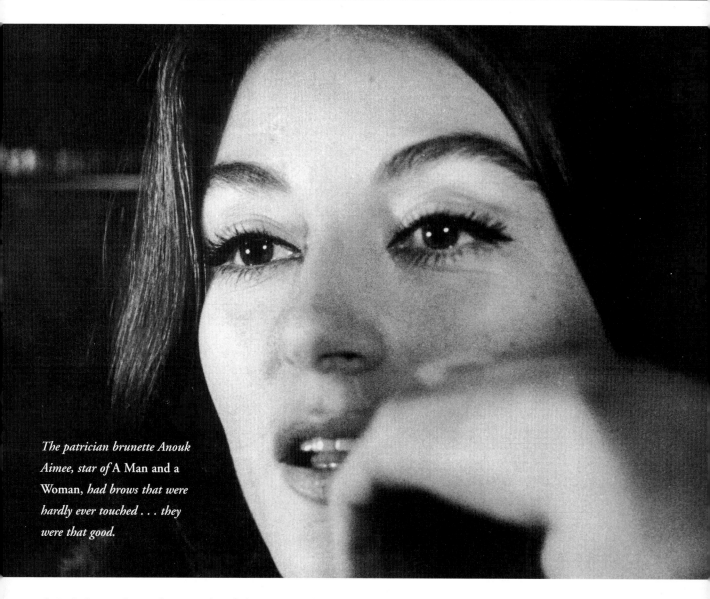

The patrician brunette Anouk Aimee, star of A Man and a Woman, *had brows that were hardly ever touched . . . they were that good.*

their disdain and apocalyptic in their fashion sense. The primary color range was black, black, and more black.

Punk may have killed disco, but what was coming would shove the Punks into the background with a heave-ho of massive shoulder pads, big hair, and bigger bank accounts. The Greed Decade was upon us.

119

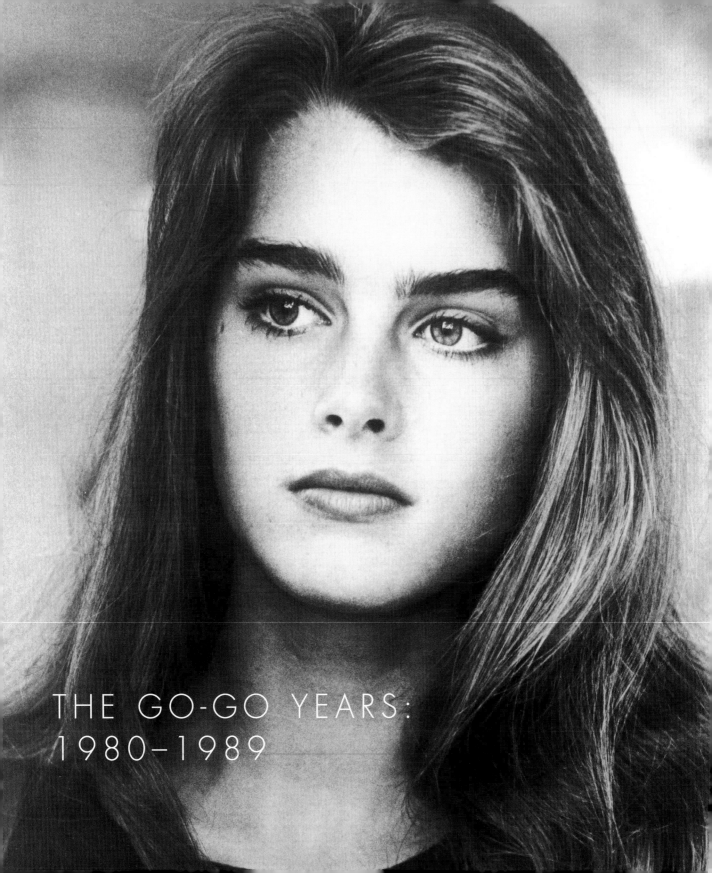

THE GO-GO YEARS:
1980–1989

When teenage model/actress Brooke Shields declared that nothing came between her and her Calvins, her thick, luxuriant eyebrows glowered sexily, and a trend was born. Models like Margaux Hemingway, Isabella Rossellini, and the curvaceous Cindy Crawford were celebrated for their expansive, expressive eyebrows. A little-known model with long, dark hair and doe eyes named Linda Evangelista had brows that bristled with impatience.

After spending a decade or two in the doldrums, plucked down or completely ignored, the eyebrow was back and considered by an ever-growing coterie of superstar makeup artists to be a bona fide fashion accessory, as necessary as a Vuitton bag or a Gucci loafer. On the face, the eyebrow became a feature of prominence that telegraphed vigor, strength, forcefulness, and success.

Everything about the 1980s was generous and overblown. Michael Douglas as arbitrageur Gordon Gekko in Oliver Stone's *Wall Street* declared, "Greed is good," which turned out to be a mantra for the time. Bond traders made and lost fortunes. Takeover specialists with their trophy wives became the Nouvelle Society in New York, displacing Mrs. Astor's 400.

Pretty baby Brooke Shields grew up in the 1980s and started a major trend toward natural brows. Her luxuriant brows were minimally groomed and allowed to flourish in all their glory.

Modern robber barons lived in baronial splendor with museum-quality art collections, seagoing yachts, private jets, Parisian *pied-à-terres,* and wives who spent more on their clothes than the annual budget of Haiti.

The voluptuousness of the age translated into clothing and makeup. Eyebrows were gloriously thick, defined, and emphasized with generous brushing, brow pencil, and brow tamer. When you let your skinny disco brows grow out, then they had to flourish as if you'd treated them with Miracle-Gro. A tweezer was used only to keep the brow from marching over the nose or to clean out the hairs that delayed the arch; otherwise, brows grew a third bigger than they'd been the decade before.

Graphic, generous brows were needed to anchor a strong face, considering where clothing and hair styles were heading in the 1980s. This was a decade of expensive excess, of angular power suits with peplums and shoulder pads as big as Joe Montana's, of Christian Lacroix pouf dresses and Azzedine Alaïa's body-grasping Ace bandage dresses, of clunky gold status jewelry from Bulgari, of Vuitton satchels and Cartier tank watches. Brand names were worshiped. Chanel made a huge comeback, and *Dynasty's* queen bitch, Alexis Carrington, played by Joan Collins wearing Nolan Miller, set an exaggerated style for at least half the decade.

In the Eighties, as the plague of AIDS was taking fashion designers, photographers, and makeup artists, physical fitness and body redesign became

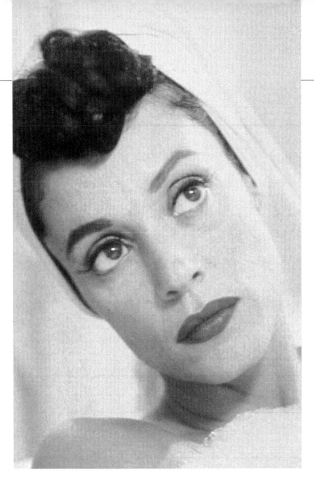

important. Jane Fonda, in yet another incarnation (she had survived *Barbarella* to become Hanoi Jane in her antiwar jeans and shag haircut), became America's workout queen. "Feel the burn" was her advice, and the overaerobicized gym rat was born. Workout chic competed with the pouf dress for supremacy as career women, happy to be out of their Thierry Mugler and Claude Montana power suits, donned Spandex tights and ripped sweatshirts (a style lifted from 1983's hit film *Flashdance),* and spent hours in the gym perfecting their abs and glutes.

The influence of professional makeup artists and fashion photographers grew in the Eighties as they created the supermodel, whose images on the covers of *Elle, Mirabella, Vogue, Bazaar, Moda,* and *Queen* were opulent, sensual, romantic, and quite overdone. Supplanting movie stars as the primary influences on the modern woman, the supermodel's every move was clocked by the paparazzi and the gossip columnist. She became the trophy amour of rock star, millionaire, and sports figure alike.

In 1987, Linda Evangelista, who once stated she wouldn't get out of bed for anything less than $10,000, was taken in hand by photographer Steven Meisel and totally redone. He said in *Allure,* "I saw her wide nose, full cheeks and weak chin . . . we went into the makeup room and began surgery." First, Meisel had Evangelista's brows tweezed, thinning and shaping them into a contemporary rendering of the 1950s brow—Diva Arch and all. He turned her into a chameleon who changed her hair at whim. When the sultry brunette went bright red, so did her brows.

No Eighties icon changed more than Madonna. While Michael Jackson was trying on his friend Elizabeth Taylor's thick brows, bleaching his skin, and paring his nose down to nothing, Madonna was performing a type of surgery on herself. Bursting out of the downtown New York scene early in the decade, Madonna had a raffish, ragamuffin charm in

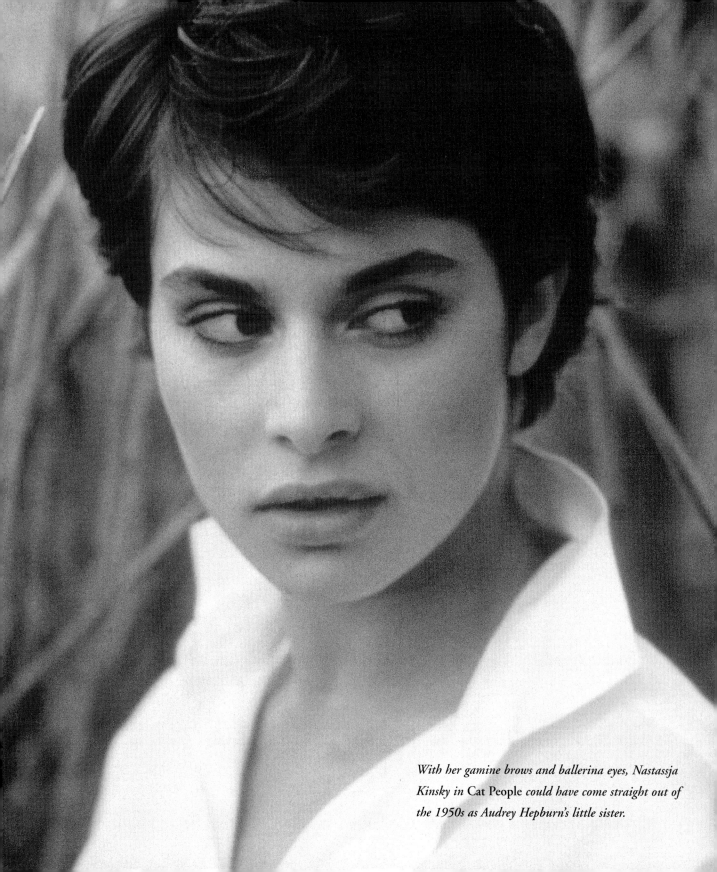

With her gamine brows and ballerina eyes, Nastassja Kinsky in Cat People *could have come straight out of the 1950s as Audrey Hepburn's little sister.*

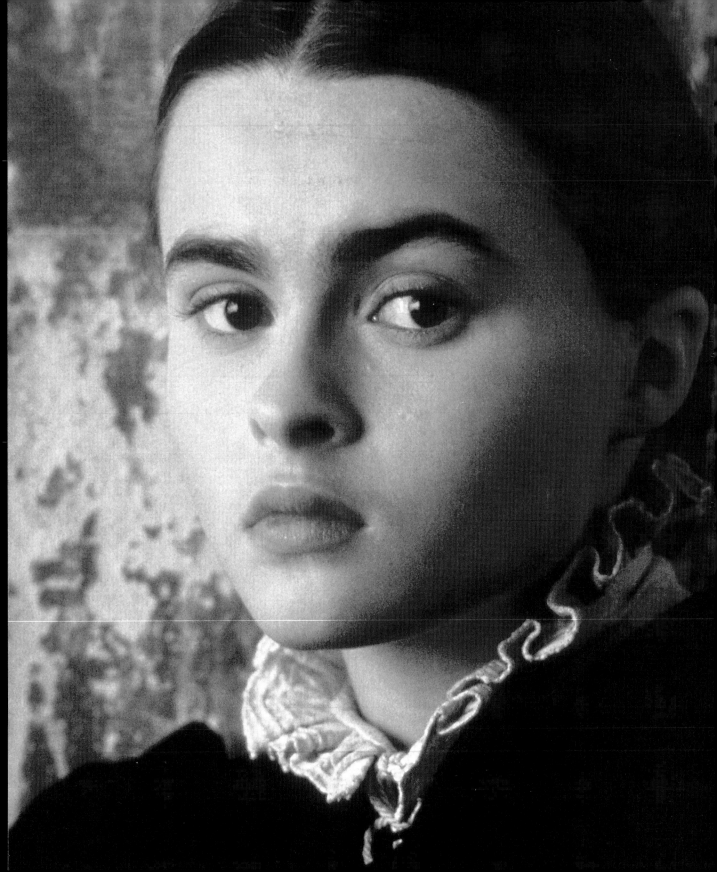

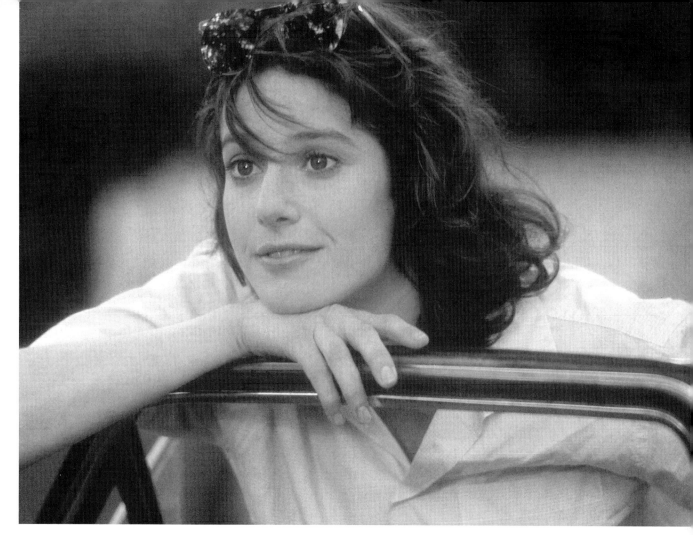

her thrift-store finery, ripped opera hose, jangly cru-
cifixes, and runaway Sicilian widow eyebrows, which
looked to be untouched by human hand or tweezer.

From the adorably cheeky rag doll of 1983, she

At the beginning of her film career, when she starred in
Lady Jane, *nineteen-year-old British ingenue Helena
Bonham-Carter had brows so thick and unruly that they
almost met over her nose. They gave her face a querulous,
angry mien, but were typical of the period when Brooke
Shields and Margaux Hemingway set the eyebrow look.*

*Debra Winger has always chosen fairly unconventional roles,
and so has never had to conform to classic Hollywood beauty
standards. She has a naturally pretty look with her tousled
dark hair, sensuous mouth, and brows that have always been
perfectly proportioned for her face—neither too thick nor too
thin. She is not the sort of woman who follows trends slavishly.*

progressed to the Material Girl, wearing innerwear as
outerwear and searching for her Boy Toys. Her brows
were on their way down, but they were still fairly
thick and black, although a forest of teensy hairs,

125

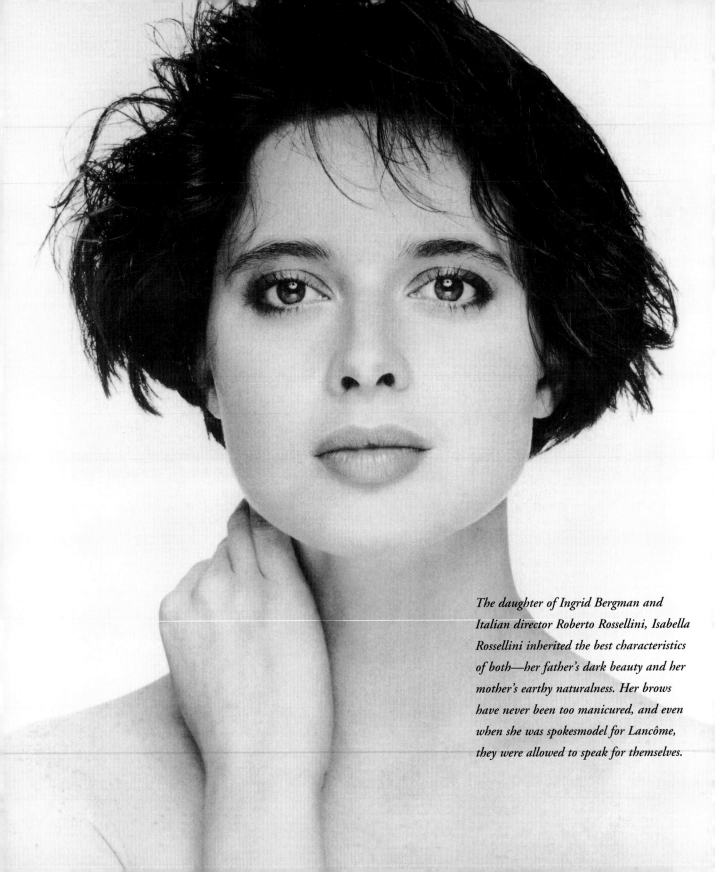

*The daughter of Ingrid Bergman and
Italian director Roberto Rossellini, Isabella
Rossellini inherited the best characteristics
of both—her father's dark beauty and her
mother's earthy naturalness. Her brows
have never been too manicured, and even
when she was spokesmodel for Lancôme,
they were allowed to speak for themselves.*

Playing opposite Tom Cruise in Top Gun, *Kelly McGillis sported the thick, out-of-control eyebrow of the Eighties.*

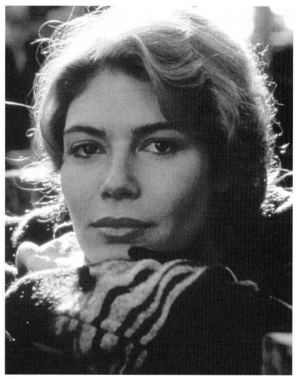

support struts, had been waxed away. By the time she toured the country in her outrageous pointy-bra costumes designed by Jean-Paul Gaultier, she had cut her hair and dyed it platinum, trained her body into gristly firmness, and groomed her brows in proper proportion to her features, which were, by all standards, quite delicate and pretty. Her eyebrows got even smaller when she exhorted drag queen and gay boy alike to "strike a pose." Her brows came off almost completely when she was cast as Eva Perón in *Evita*, but as a new mother in

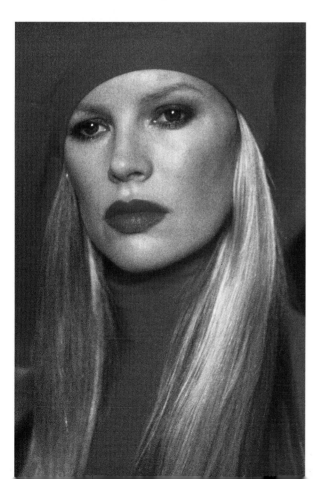

1995, she softened her image with fuller brows and strawberry blond hair.

The Eighties' brow was cared for like a stock portfolio and investment jewelry. In a growing number of destination and day spas, you could get your eyebrows waxed, tweezed, dyed, and even tattooed. On both face and body, what nature had stinted upon could also be augmented by plastic surgery. Tired, fading

In My Stepmother Was an Alien, *former model Kim Basinger, a blonde so pale that her own brows don't show up, wore nicely defined brows that had been emphasized with brown brow powder.*

127

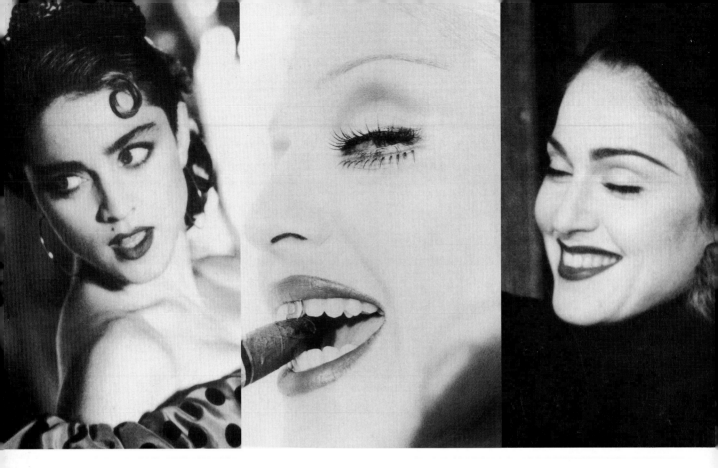

beauty could be freshened up by cosmetic surgery, drooping lids and wrinkled brows could be lifted by endoscopic brow surgery, and sagging or nonexistent breasts suddenly became huge . . . quite obvious with the development of the silicone breast implant.

The tattooing fad extended not only from the eyebrows with minuscule vertical "hairs" painstakingly traced on by needle, but to lips and permanent eyeliner. Ostensibly, tattooing eliminated the need for brow pencil, eyeliner, and lipstick. But the colors faded, minds changed, and the fad receded.

The signature makeup look in the late 1980s came from M.A.C, a Canadian company founded by a makeup artist, one of the first of the so-called lim-

ited-distribution artistry lines that have flourished ever since. Foundation was matte and had a tawny or yellowish cast. Lips were deep brown or burgundy, almost liverish-looking, and matte-finished. Madonna preferred M.A.C's Russian Red, and Viva Glam, a deep burgundy, whose sales were donated to AIDS charities, became a classic. There was, however, a huge emphasis on having the perfect brow, and every makeup artist, before he or she even began to paint a face, groomed or restyled the eyebrows. Brows were thick and designed. They carried the face. Eyes were lined slightly and then smudged over beige or neutral shadow. It was a face of all brows and mouth. And it was soon to change radically.

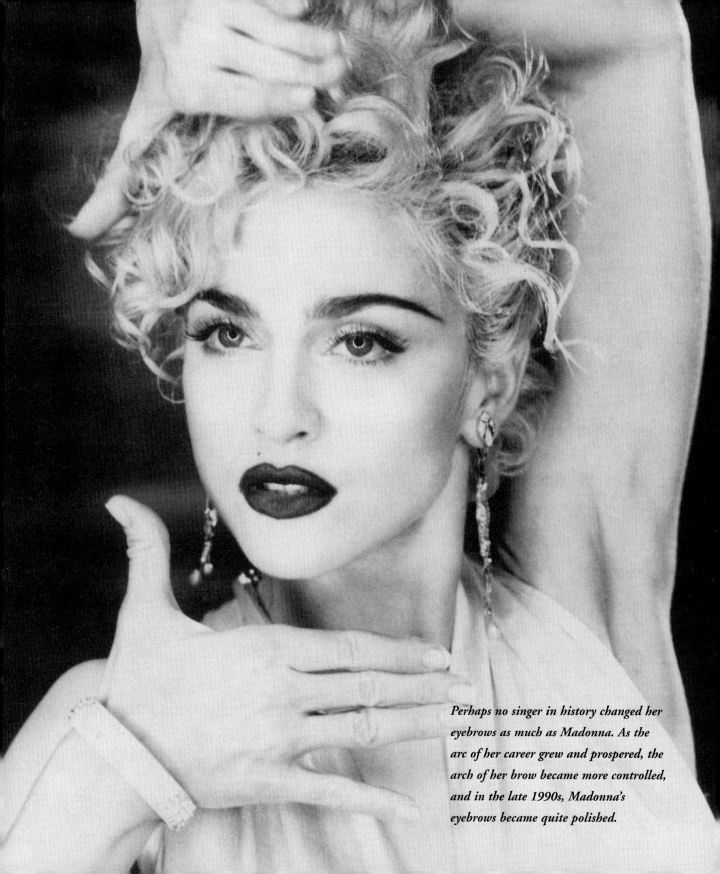

Perhaps no singer in history changed her eyebrows as much as Madonna. As the arc of her career grew and prospered, the arch of her brow became more controlled, and in the late 1990s, Madonna's eyebrows became quite polished.

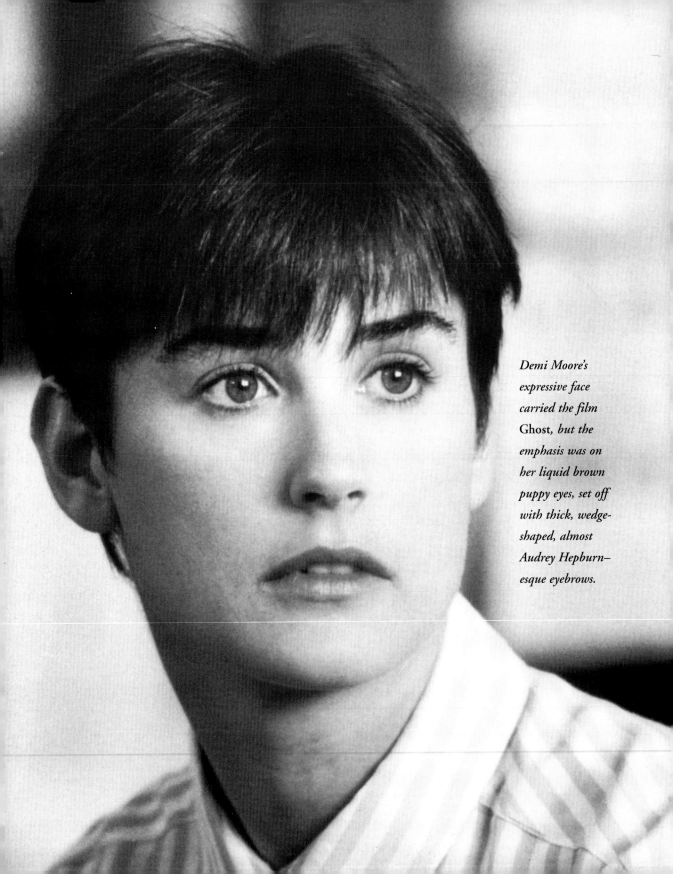

Demi Moore's expressive face carried the film Ghost, *but the emphasis was on her liquid brown puppy eyes, set off with thick, wedge-shaped, almost Audrey Hepburn—esque eyebrows.*

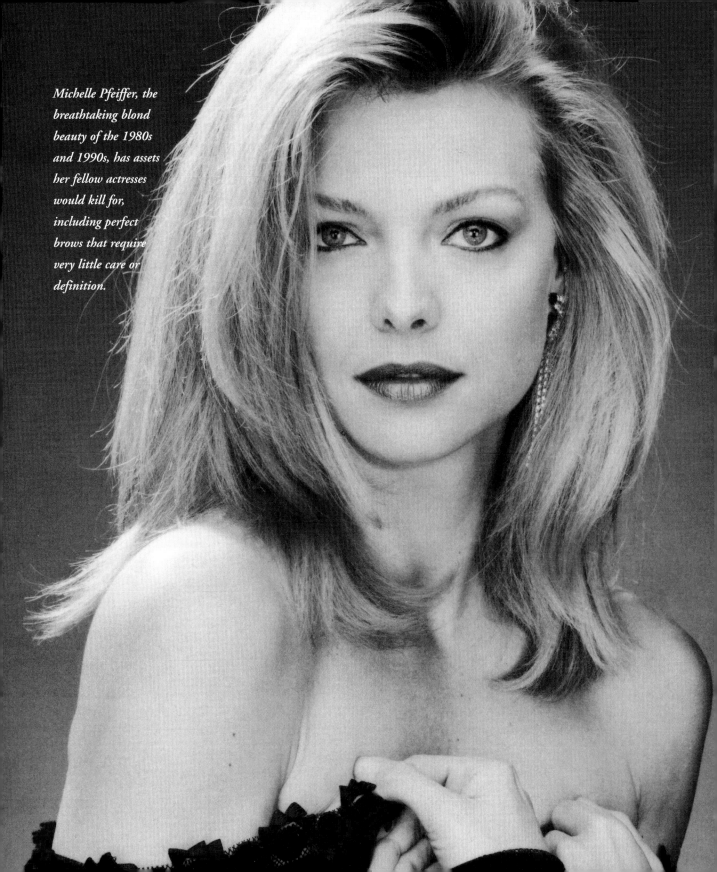

Michelle Pfeiffer, the breathtaking blond beauty of the 1980s and 1990s, has assets her fellow actresses would kill for, including perfect brows that require very little care or definition.

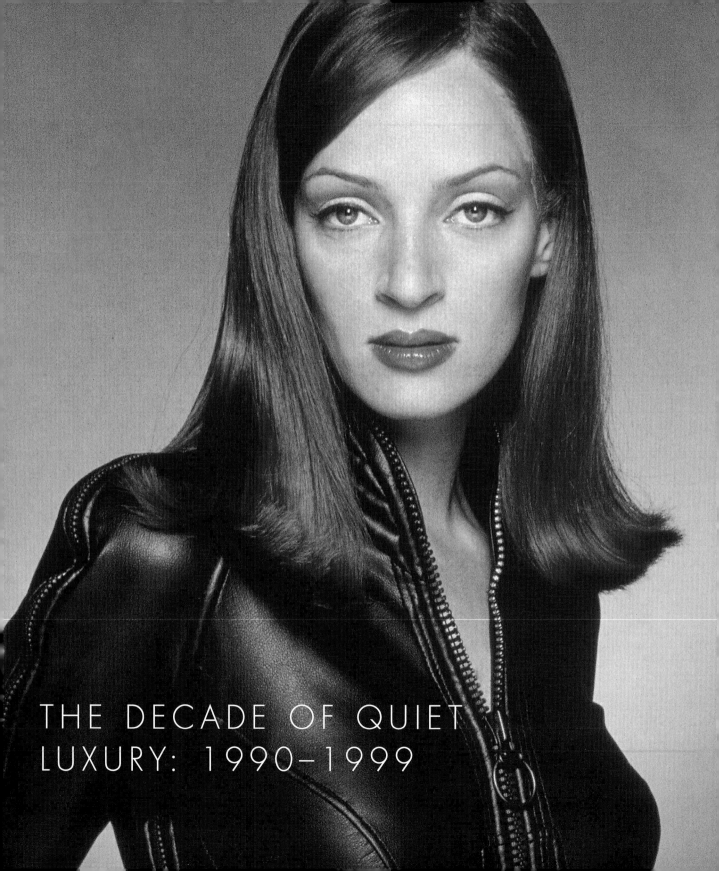

THE DECADE OF QUIET
LUXURY: 1990–1999

At the start of the 1990s, the American woman was still getting her fashion cues from the front covers of slick magazines, and the news was not good. The fashion editors were worshiping the Waif, a birdlike critter who was younger, scrawnier, more boyish, and definitely wore less makeup than in the previous ten years. In a total reaction to the excesses of the Eighties, the new decade, in what was nearly an antifashion mode, began with a giant step backward to retrench, relax, and regroup.

In the opening years of the last decade of the millennium, conspicuous consumption went underground. But quality didn't. If anything, the yearning for luxury increased. It just got quieter and more discreet. The limousine culture reverted to subtler town cars and sedans; clothes became simpler, with an emphasis on linear separates, clean lines, a dearth of decoration, and dark, somber colors. Designers like Calvin Klein and Donna Karan used a limited palette of black, black, and more black. Luxury was in the fabrication, not the decoration.

As Punk settled into smaller and smaller enclaves, a new down-to-earth, common-man sensibility overtook the country as Seattle grunge rockers exported their flannel shirt chic to the rest of the country. The Waif was emblematic of this pared-down sensibility. She was a girl creature who looked barely old enough to take a history final, let alone support *haute couture* on a Parisian runway. The healthy, voluptuous supermodels—Cindy Crawford, Christie Brinkley, and Linda Evangelista—moved over for their younger, skinnier, and more gaunt sisters. Kate Moss was the prototype.

New York makeup artists Dick Page and Kevyn Aucoin designed the looks for most of the cover models. Because the Waif was so young and fresh, Page eliminated foundation altogether, mixed lipstick with Vaseline to tint the cheeks, slid Vaseline onto the eyelid, and used a minimal amount of mascara. Kate Moss's eyebrows were scant and feathery, and Page groomed them with a bit of brow fix but otherwise ignored them. Aucoin and photographer Steven Meisel often worked in tandem on models like Moss, Amber Valetta, Christy Turlington, and Naomi Campbell. Aucoin played with eyebrows. In his 1994 book *The Art of Makeup*, he said, "To me, the eyebrows are the most important feature on the face. They're the most expressive feature, as well as the one that can be changed the most drastically without cosmetic surgery." And change the brow he did.

He redesigned it and he dyed it. The Aucoin brow was arched, but not as high or as prominent as the Diva Arch of the 1950s. He accomplished his brow makeovers by brushing the brows straight up and then toward the hairline with a small eyebrow

As the modern-day version of Diana Rigg's Emma Peel in The Avengers, *Uma Thurman wore a true Diva brow— tweezed, darkened, and haughty.*

The only Hollywood [star]
who can get away w[ith]
having no eyebrows
is Oscar-winner Wh[oopi]
Goldberg.

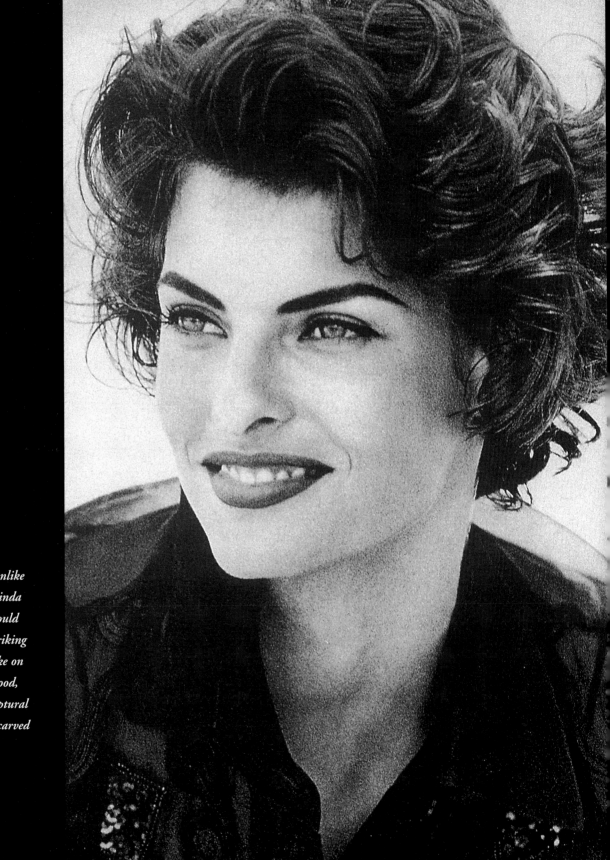

The chameleonlike supermodel Linda Evangelista could change her striking features to take on Fifties Divahood, from her sculptural brows to her carved lipline.

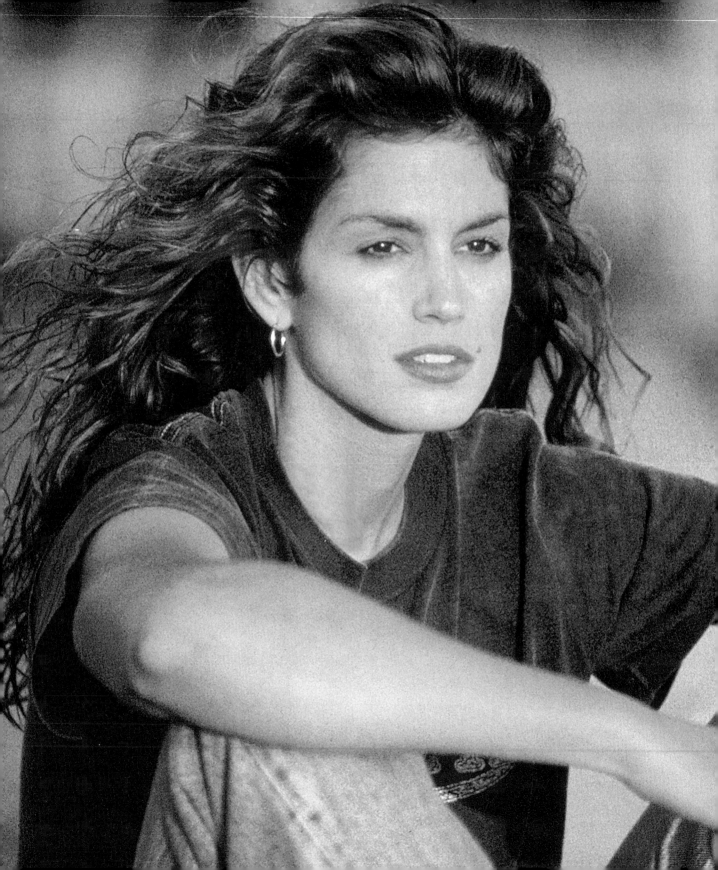

Starting in the 1980s, Cindy Crawford, one of the first bona fide supermodels, wore her eyebrows to reflect the fad of the moment. Her best look came in the mid-Nineties, when she thinned her brows a bit and groomed them into a gentle, slightly elongated arch that opened up her face under her dark chestnut hair.

brush, which he deemed "one of the most under-used and under-appreciated make up tools. It is essential because simply brushing the eyebrows upward can open up the eye area and reveal the hairs that need tweezing." To accomplish his ideal brow, Aucoin blocked out the offending hairs with white liner pencil and plucked away. His brow was very distinctive and it worked on the pared-down face, giving his already genetically blessed model clients a wide-eyed, little-girl-lost look.

But when he began bleaching brows, the models he worked with took on an otherworldly, alien appearance. For a *Vogue* layout, he bleached Christy Turlington's eyebrows down to a light golden blond to match the blond wig she wore, and focused solely on her exquisite lips, which he enlarged with liner and painted in with carmine lipstick. The brows were so pale, they looked like sunspots on her forehead. He made the statuesque Nadja Auermann's

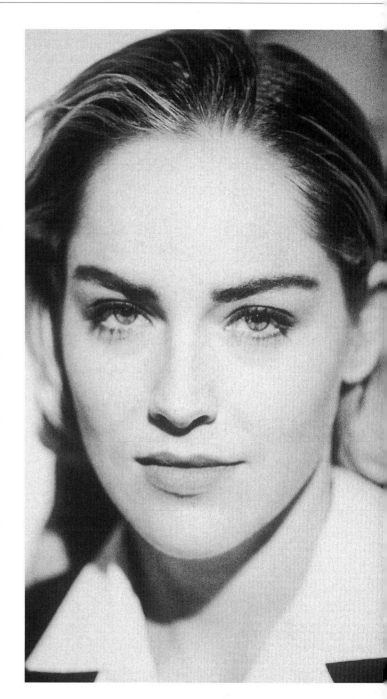

On the brink of superstardom after Basic Instinct, *Sharon Stone became one of Hollywood's true glamour girls, with her red-red lips and goddess eyebrows—brows to kill for.*

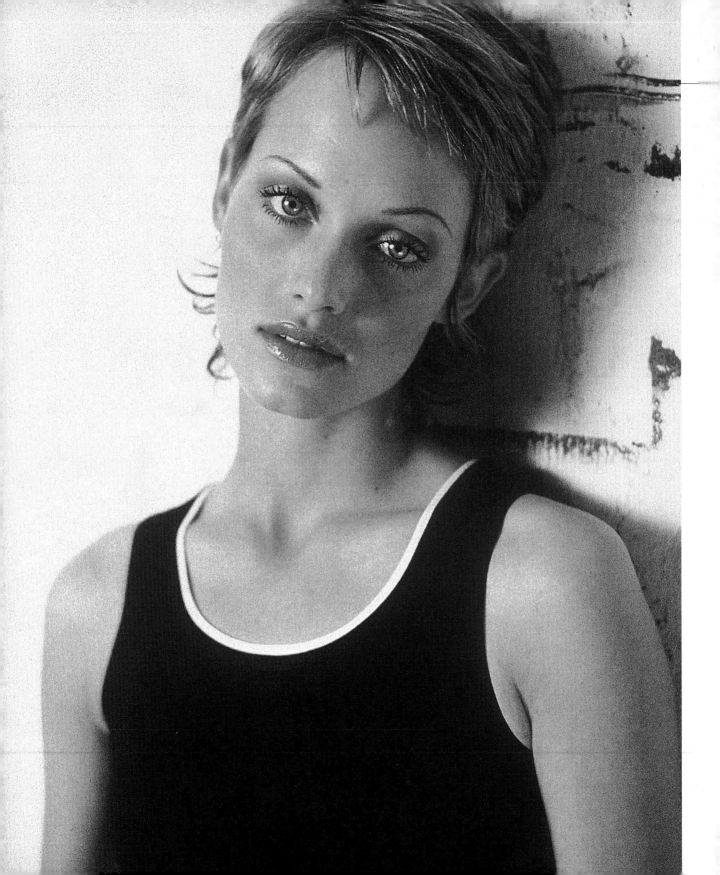

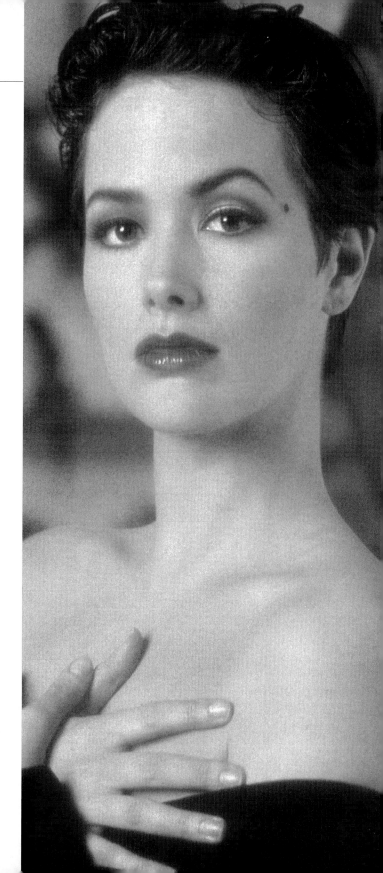

In the early 1990s, Waifs like Amber Valetta became the favorite image of fashion magazines and photographers such as Steven Meisel. It was like photographing prepubescent teenagers. Makeups were almost nonexistent, and eyebrows were as thin as their owners. It was an ugly time for women with curvy bodies and thick brows.

brows such a light blond that they almost disappeared. Auermann's cropped hair was platinum then, and her eyes were exaggerated pools of heavy black liner and fake lashes. The effect was stunning. There were times, however, when the extreme tweezing, tinting, bleaching, and obliteration of the brow (model Kristin McMenamy shaved hers off altogether) prompted a model to disappear on an extended vacation until her eyebrows grew back.

Most of Aucoin's model makeovers in the early 1990s were a huge improvement over the comparatively garish makeups of the 1980s. He brought a new subtlety and a lighter hand that enhanced rather than overrode his subject's natural endowments. For instance, he thinned Cindy Crawford's abundant arch and slanted it more toward her nose, although he still kept her brows wide set. Uniformly

Northern Exposure*'s* Janine Turner *may have played an Alaskan bush pilot in checkered shirts and Timberland boots, but her brunette good looks and direct gaze were anchored by film goddess brows.*

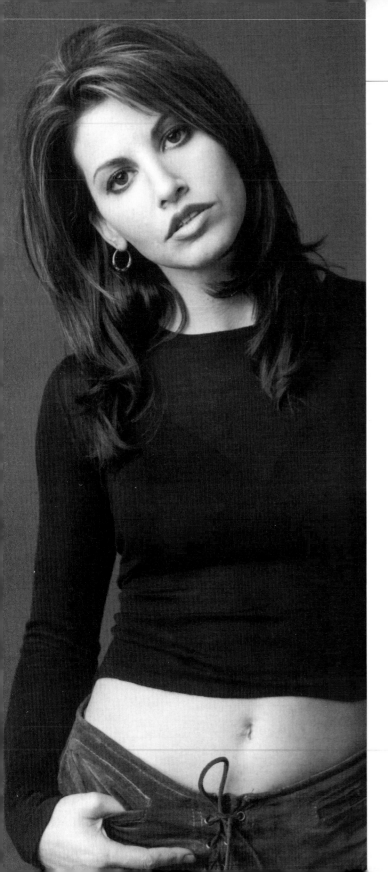

brown, the brows were brushed into shape and anchored with brow gel.

Soon the press and the public tired of the scrawny Waif, but she lingered on and became transmogrified into an even unhealthier look—heroin chic, a bony girl with lank hair and a dark, moody face with ghostly eyes, tweezed-down brows, and a cloudy complexion. One of the few models who swam against that current was Linda Evangelista, whose haughty face had brows and lips lifted straight out of the 1950s. Her lips, eyes, nose, and hands were the only things to appear on the front cover of the Fabian Baron *Harper's Bazaar* redesign. Her brows had been arched as if they belonged to Lisa Fonssagrieves, and her lips were bright red and carved with definition.

By the mid-Nineties, the cult of the makeup artist had trickled down to the cosmetics counter as more and more New York makeup professionals fielded their own commercial lines. The fashion designer and the person who designed the runway look set a fast pace for the face. Every year or so, the

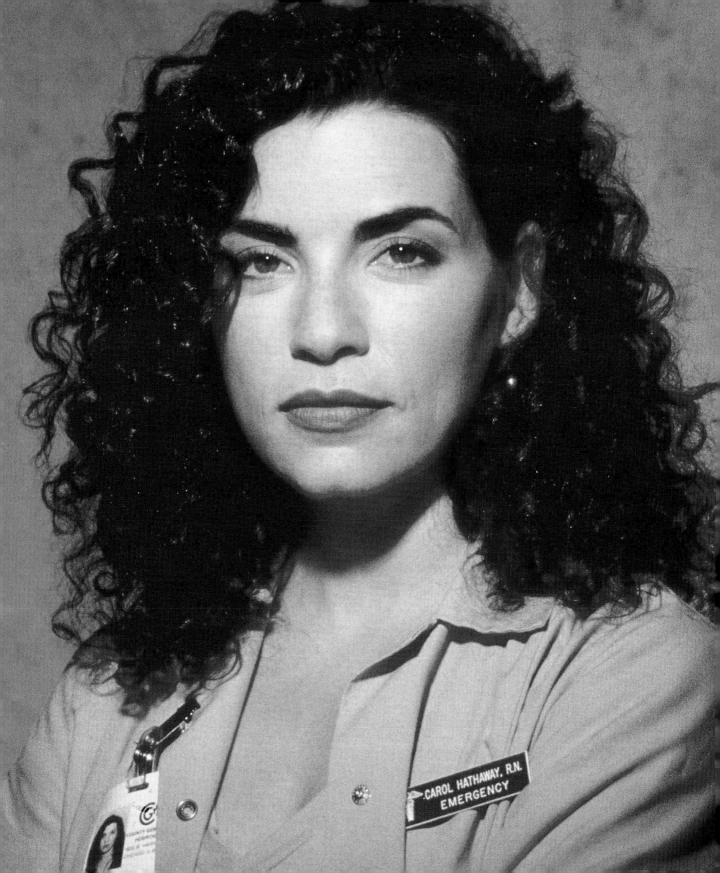

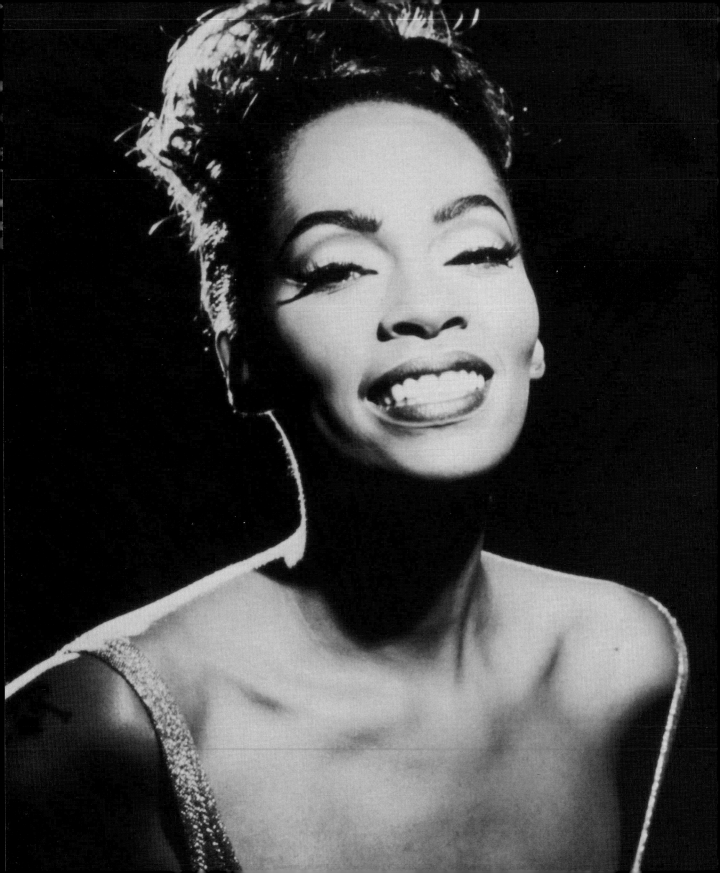

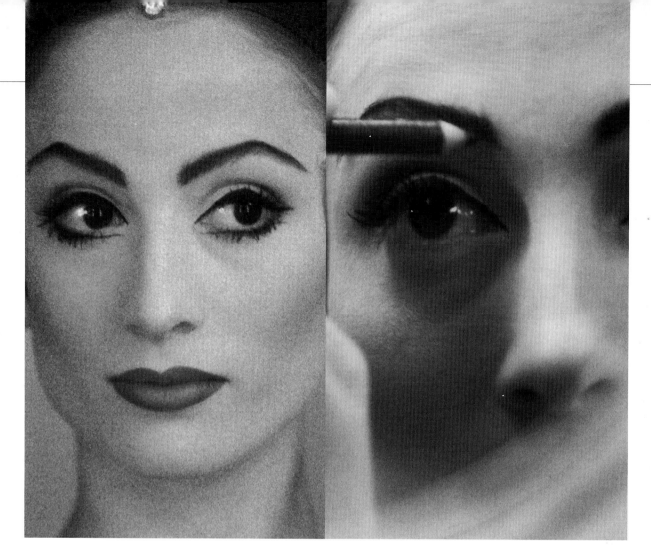

look changed. Trish McEvoy, Bobbi Brown, Laura Mercier, and François Nars designed neutral faces that required a lot of makeup to look natural. The mid-Nineties face belonged to rose-brown lip glosses, sheer blush, and lightly made-up eyes. Faces were out-and-out lovely, not plastic. If a model had great brows, they were left pretty much alone; superfluous

Jody Watley's naturally elegant eyebrows are as expressive as her singing style.

Beautiful Julie Kent, a prima ballerina with the American Ballet Theatre, wears traditional ballet eye makeup. Note that it doesn't look much different from Dame Margot Fonteyn's, decades later.

hairs were taken out with a tweezer and brows were brushed into place with brow tamer.

As the decade grew older, music, film, and TV stars began exerting their influence on fashion and beauty. No one had better or more perfect brows

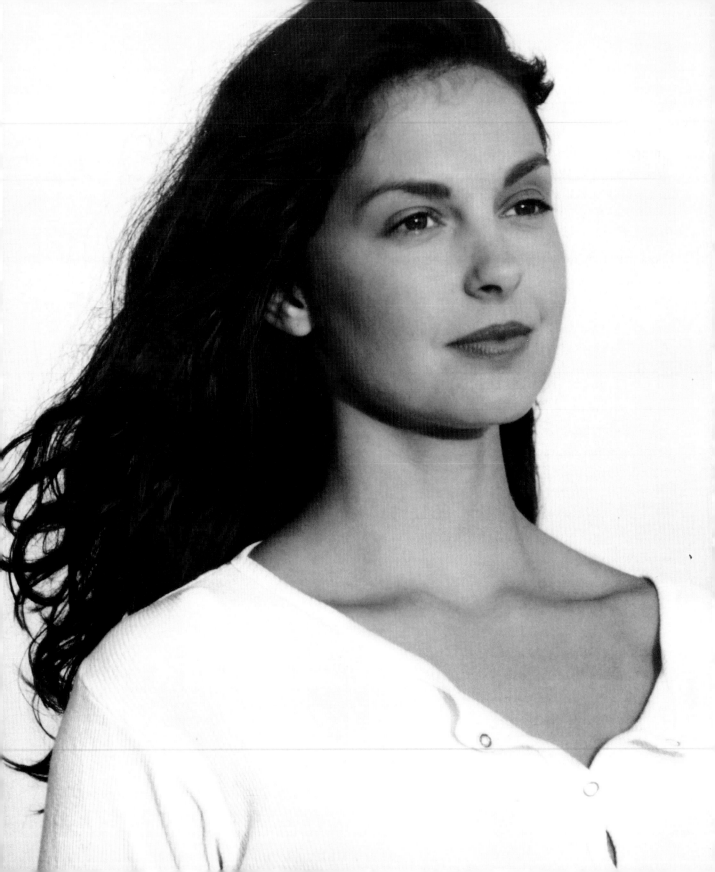

than Sharon Stone, Michelle Pfeiffer, Angie Harmon, or Teri Hatcher—each and every one a timeless beauty blessed with a natural arch, huge eyes, and perfect skin. Stone's well-manicured dark brows worked well with her steady gaze and her *fin-de-siècle* short, spiky hairdo for *The Muse*. With some judicious tweezing, Hatcher went from Girl-Next-Door parts as Lois Lane in television's *Lois and Clark* to Femme Fatale status in the James Bond film with Pierce Brosnan, *Tomorrow Never Dies*.

In the remaining years of the decade, the eyebrow once again became as iconic as it had been in the 1950s, due in part to the retro nature of *fin-de-siècle* fashion and also the influence of three fashion designers. Todd Oldham started the trend toward fuller, darker brows when he pasted black plastic brows over his runway models' natural eyebrows. Gucci's Tom Ford harkened back to the 1970s Italian fashion model and the stylized photography of Helmut Newton when he designed an eye that was all smoke, liner, and double fake lashes under a narrow and defined brow. And when Karl Lagerfeld sent models down his fall 1999 Chanel runway in Paris, they wore smudgy, rode-hard-and-put-up-wet eyes. He told his makeup designers that he

One of the most elegant of the millennial actresses of Hollywood, Ashley Judd is a classic beauty with a pair of brows so precisely groomed they would be quite at home in the 1950s.

wanted the girls to look as if they'd been up all night partying. The brows, however, were beautifully designed, neat and dark.

In the Nineties, the prominence of a well-groomed brow returned. Every major cosmetics company designed an eyebrow kit with brush, tweezer, and definer in a variety of colors aimed at matching the exact tone of a brow. Acceptance of plastic surgery to enhance and correct became a norm. Botox, or botulism toxin, which is injected between the brows, works on relaxing the muscles that cause horizontal creases and the stress-induced, vertical "11s" between the eyes. The result is a clear, perfect forehead and wide-set brows, ready for enhancement.

There are, as in every decade, the stylistic rebels, and in the 1990s, a small but visually arresting population of modern primitives continued the iconographic attitudes and attire of radical Punk and Sadomasochistic movements, affecting black leather, truncheonlike boots, shaved and/or tattooed heads, and body modifications. In the artistic and gay communities, there were coteries of men and women who used their bodies as ongoing art projects, celebrating every life passage—a birthday, a divorce, a new relationship, a move to another city, or a psychological milestone—by tattooing themselves with graphic black-work designs, Maori-style inkwork, or elaborate Japanese-style color work that could

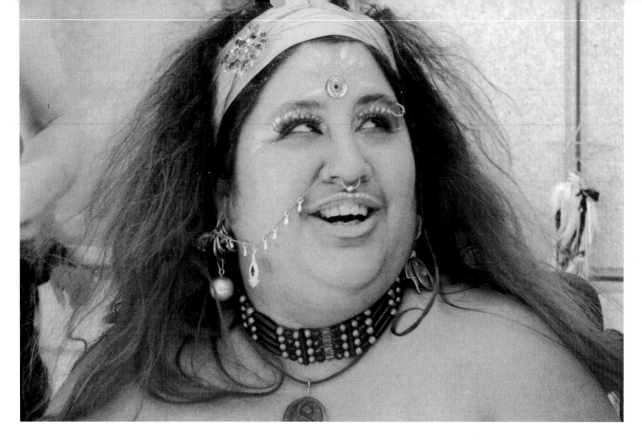

Wolfie's face is painted with traditional Indian designs; her nose is pierced in two places; and she wears a delicate silver eyebrow ring.

encompass an entire back; scarring or branding their bodies with white-hot irons; and body piercings.

Not restricted to earlobes, any body part or protrusion could be pierced, including noses, navels, nipples, genitals, and eyebrows. Eyebrow piercings were done with sterile needles of 18- or 14-gauge, depending upon the size of the jewelry inserted in the brow. Eyebrows could be affixed with delicate steel or silver rings, chrome barbells, or colorful titanium spikes. Accomplished with a minimum of pain (a hard pinch, more than anything else), eyebrow piercings heal in about two or three months. Eventually, the body will reject the piercing, although for some people, the process could take years.

The march of the eyebrow through the twentieth century has landed it in a prominent spot. As necessary an embellishment and accoutrement as a Prada bag or a pair of diamond studs, the eyebrow—a renewable resource if cared for gently—is now classic, manicured to perfection, and geared solely for the face on which it sits.

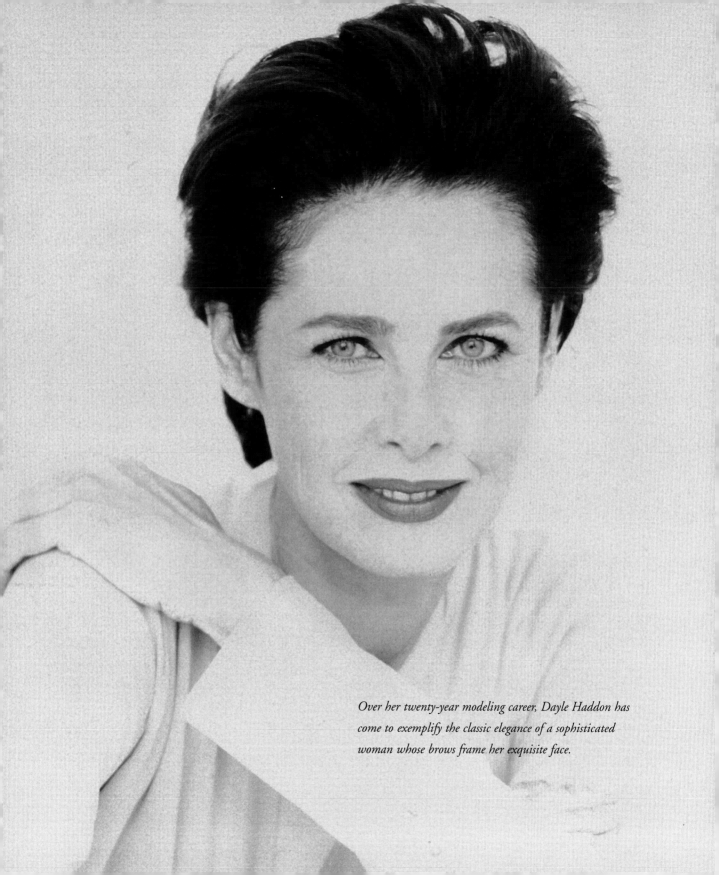

Over her twenty-year modeling career, Dayle Haddon has come to exemplify the classic elegance of a sophisticated woman whose brows frame her exquisite face.

WHOSE BROWS ARE THESE?

Throughout the twentieth century, there have been women who have had eyebrows that have personalities all their own. Just for fun, I'd like to test your Brow-Q. Who are these women? For the correct answers, turn the page.

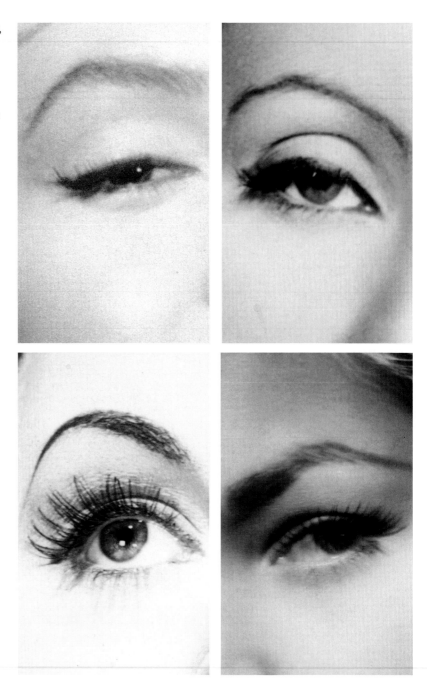

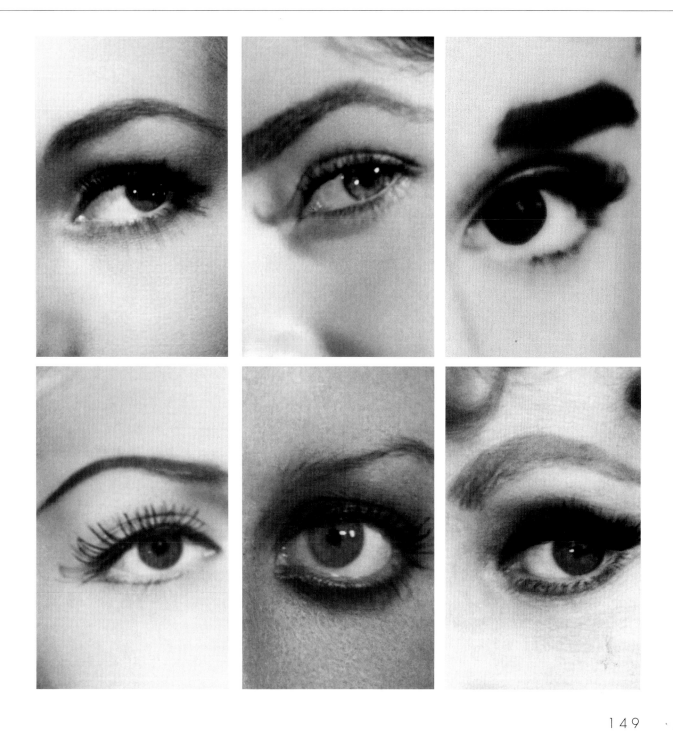

WHOSE BROWS ARE THESE?

Marilyn Monroe
Greta Garbo
Kim Novak
Elizabeth Taylor
Audrey Hepburn

Hedy Lamarr
Lauren Bacall
Lana Turner
Joan Crawford
Lucille Ball

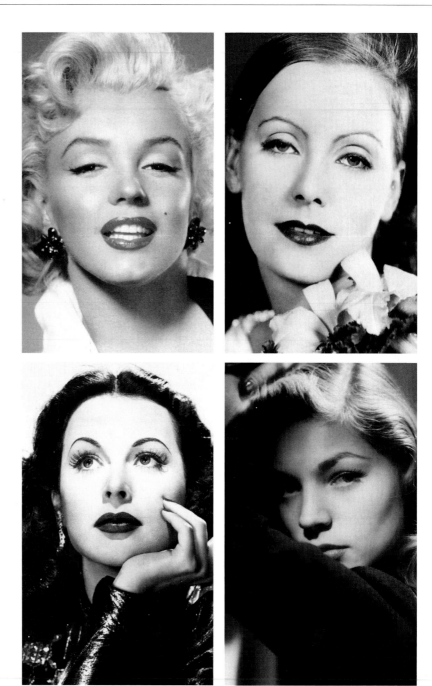

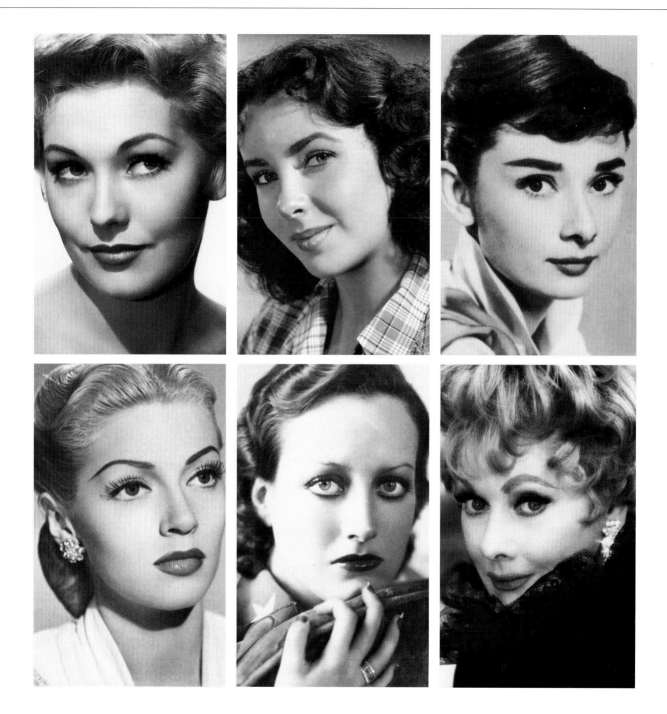

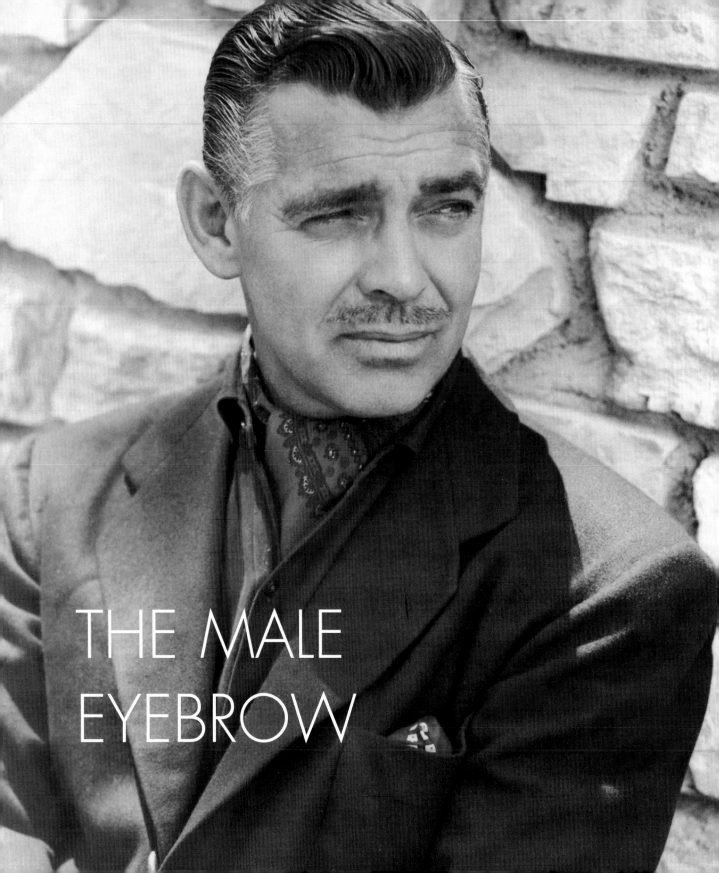

THE MALE
EYEBROW

t's safe to say that most human beings have eyebrows. But some people's eyebrows are created more distinctive than others—so distinctive that even without the rest of the face, if you know the eyebrow, you know the person.

So far, it's been the women who have held center stage, and as we've seen, they are aces at manipulating, coloring, tweezing, and otherwise changing their eyebrows. In the process, they change their attitude, their look, and often, as in the case of actresses such as Joan Crawford or Marlene Dietrich, the entire direction of their careers. But men . . . well, men are different. Very few men will mess with their eyebrows. And what they see in the mirror is usually what you'll see on their faces.

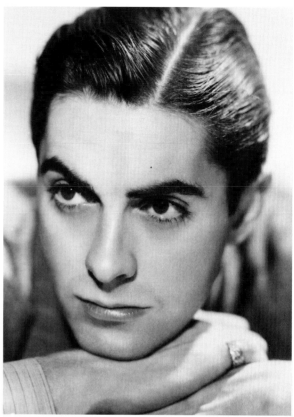

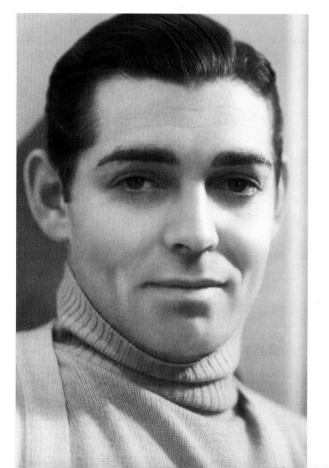

It has only been in the last decade that some men have tended to their eyebrows, going to facial salons or spas and, in a private room, having an esthetician or brow expert tweeze out hairs that march across their noses, or even tinting their brows to make them look thicker.

A man and his brows are so closely identified that it seems either the man takes on the personality of the brow or the eyebrow has adapted itself to the personality of the

OPPOSITE AND LEFT: *Clark Gable, older and younger*
ABOVE: *Tyrone Power*

153

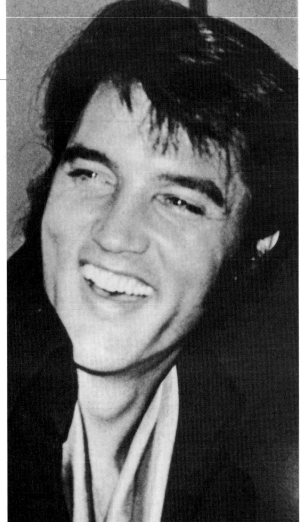

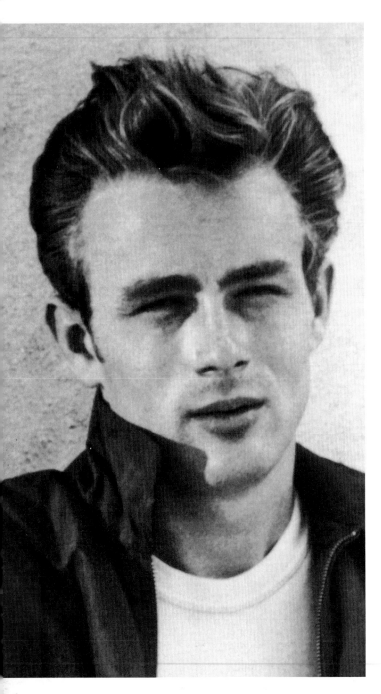

man. What would Clint Eastwood be without his sun-bleached, heavily knitted brows? Could *Dirty Harry* have ever been so menacing if Eastwood's brows hadn't almost met above his nose in a frown—created, of course, by staring down the barrel of a .45 Magnum?

Part of the charm of the Fifties' teen idols James

LEFT: *James Dean*

ABOVE: *Elvis Presley*

OPPOSITE: *Clint Eastwood, Sean Connery*

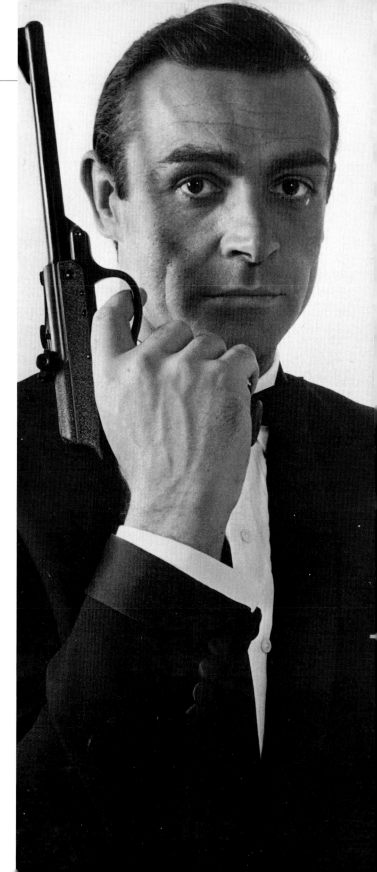

Dean and Elvis Presley was eyebrows so black, thick, and expressive, they could make a teenager swoon. Presley's brows looked inky compared to his naturally brown hair, but as his career advanced, his hair darkened, and by the time he made his comeback appearances in Las Vegas, both his eyebrows and his hair were as black as boot polish. As for Dean, his sleepy-eyed look—so evident in *Rebel Without a Cause* and *Giant*—would never have been the same had his brows not been so straight and dense. They gave his face an air of defi-

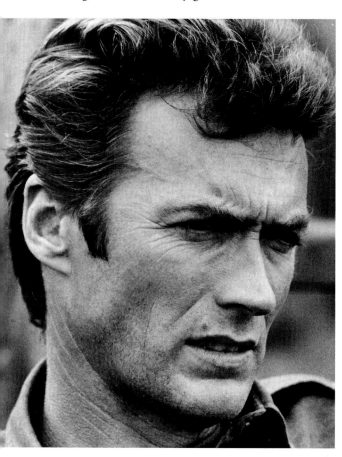

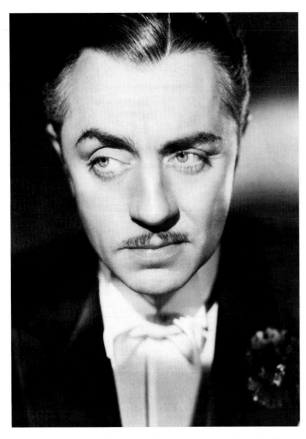

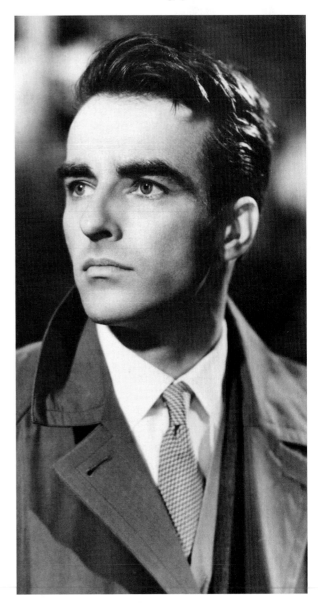

ance and anger that was mitigated only by the hurt puppy look in his eyes. An irresistible combination.

In the 1940s and 1950s, matinee idols such as Montgomery Clift, Tyrone Power, William Powell, Clark Gable, and Humphrey Bogart mesmerized women with the directness of their gaze, framed by their magnificent brows. Powell's, Clift's, and Power's arched so naturally that they could have been the envy of arch-deficient women. Theirs were the male equivalent of the Diva Arch. As for Bogart, his brows were so full and masculine that his forthright directness—so

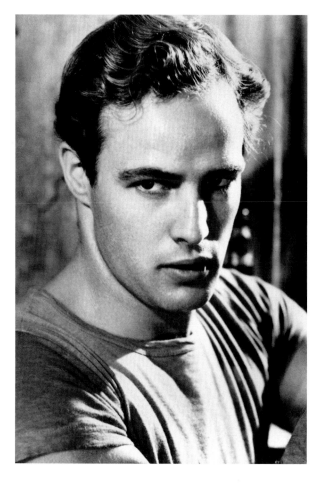

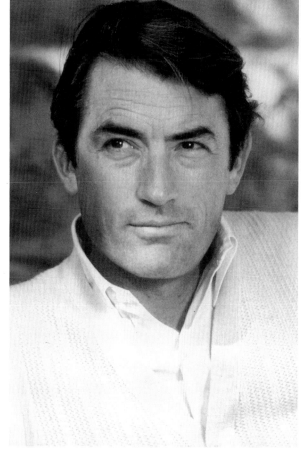

attractive and interpreted as "tough"—masked the tender aspects of his film characterizations. Other movie idols captured the hearts of film fans because their expressive eyes and brows connoted deep, unspoken emotion. Marlon Brando's signature eyebrow scar in *On the Waterfront* was a clue to the vulnerability of his character, Terry. Sean Connery's fierce Scottish brows, which he could arch or wiggle at will, cemented James Bond's martini-dry British understatement. For singu-

lar beauty, there are the puppy-dog eyes of Gregory Peck, masculinized by thick, elegantly shaped brows. And the same goes for Al Pacino, whose Italianate good looks start at his licorice-black eyebrows and proceed down his aquiline face.

Sir Laurence Olivier became one of Hollywood's best character actors as he aged. His classically carved features—sometimes his face looked as if it could have been struck from an ancient Greek coin—were

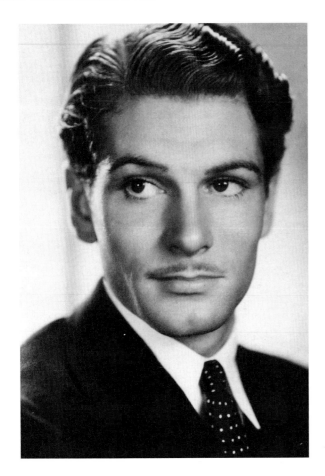

perfect foils as his character in *The Shining* went bonkers. And as the Devil incarnate in *The Witches of Eastwick,* he didn't have to do much more than wiggle his eyebrows to get into character. Nicholson's brows can get very physical, as they did in *As Good As It Gets.* Then there was Boris Karloff, the classic Forties' horror star, who had heavy, oppressive brows, which added to the menace of the roles he chose. For Leonard Nimoy, less was more as his own natural brows were blocked out and his Vulcan eyebrows were

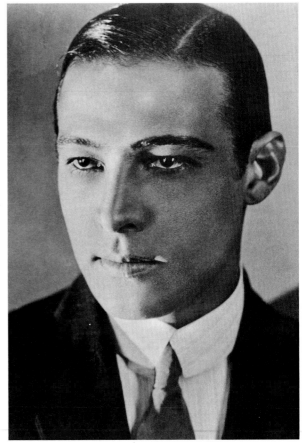

punctuated by perfectly symmetrical brows. Olivier was the kind of actor whose characterizations took life as he put them on from the outside. For *Othello,* for instance, he painted himself up in dark body and face makeup and added a curly black wig and false eyebrows before he felt comfortable in the classic Shakespearean role.

There are those fortunate actors who are blessed with eyebrows that helped define what kinds of roles they played. Jack Nicholson's devilish brows were the

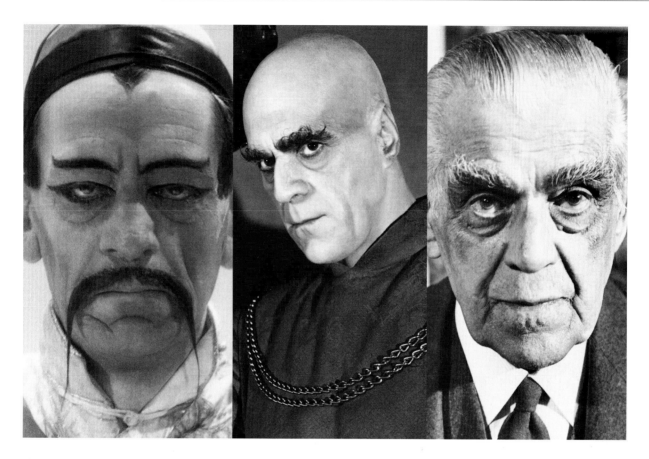

drawn on for *Star Trek*. Rudolph Valentino, Charlie Chaplin, Groucho Marx, and Yul Brynner all had brows that were manipulated for performance. And World Wrestling Federation superstar The Rock's signature is the tweezed, arched brow known as the People's Eyebrow.

Have you ever noticed that dictators, politicians, and millionaires often have something in common? Forceful, unforgettable eyebrows. Examples: Russian dictator Joseph Stalin, American labor leader John L. Lewis, Greek shipping tycoon Aristotle Onassis, and the publicity-seeking New York real estate mogul, Donald Trump. A man does not have to rule a country or build casinos or oil tankers, however, to have charismatic eyebrows. Take Gene Shalit, the film critic for NBC's *Today*. Above his tinted aviator glasses, his eyebrows definitely hold their own.

When is a guy not a guy? When he is in drag, whether it is female attire or performance costume.

OPPOSITE: *Laurence Olivier, Rudolph Valentino*
ABOVE: *The many faces of Boris Karloff*

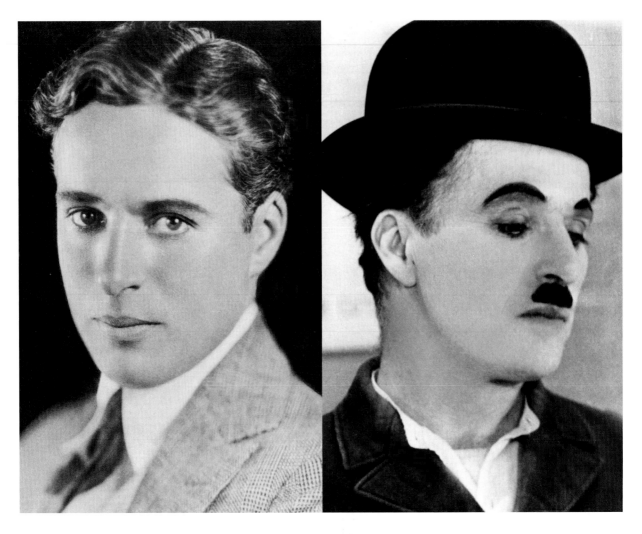

Such drag artists as Divine, Lypsinka, and RuPaul have artistically manipulated their eyebrows into an exaggeration of the feminine ideal from the 1950s. Divine, the star of many John Waters movies, had his look down. His brows were 1930s all the way—teensy, winged creatures, nearly an afterthought, that were poised to fly off his bowling-ball round face. Divine's on-screen per-

sona worked those brows like a runway model showing off Dior couture. Lypsinka's ultrafeminine brows mimic those of Joan Crawford.

Meanwhile, rock stars who have flirted with androgyny, such as David Bowie and The Artist Formerly Known as Prince (a.k.a. The Artist), are two sides of the same performance coin. As Ziggy Stardust,

OPPOSITE: *Charlie Chaplin, younger and older*
BELOW: *Groucho Marx*
RIGHT: *Yul Brynner*

the rocker space alien, Bowie dyed his hair an alarming shade of red-orange and shaved his eyebrows off completely; Prince, on the other hand, hid one of his magnificently tweezed eyebrows under a pirate's bandanna. His brows are so neatly defined and cleaned up that without viewing the rest of his face, you'd think he was a woman.

Men are not above breathtaking beauty. The male thoroughbreds are the artists of ballet, whose eyebrows and eyes are defined with black paint so they will read across the footlights. Ballet makeup is very specific: It idealizes the male face, as it did with Leonide Massine in the 1940s, Rudolf Nureyev in the 1960s, Mikhail Baryshnikov in the 1970s and early 1980s, and the

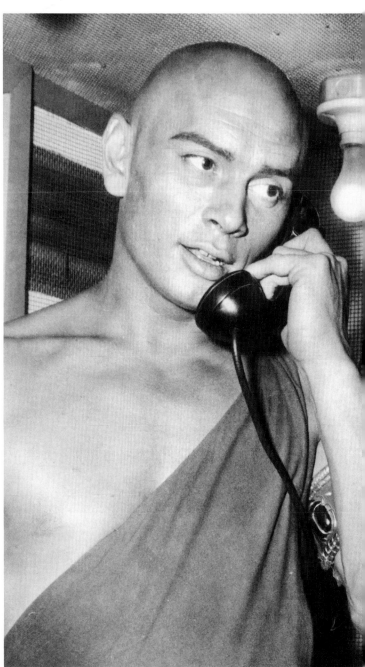

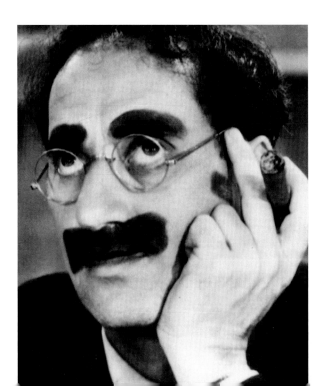

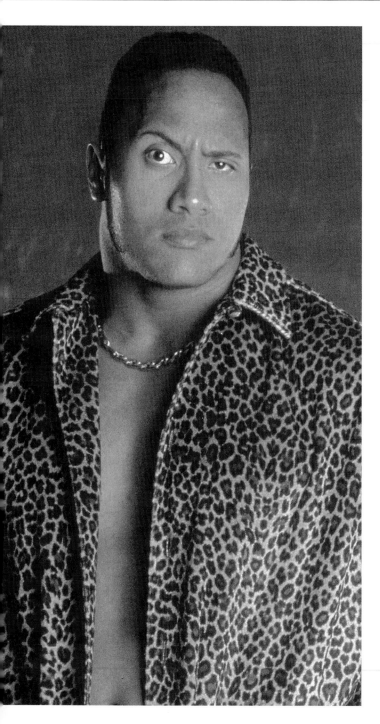

American Ballet Theatre's principal dancer of the 1990s, José Manuel Carreño.

The male dancer's eye makeup is nearly identical to his female partner's. The eye itself is defined by kohl black liner to make it look huge. The brows take their pattern from the nearly ageless icons of the Ballets Russes from the 1920s—a Mandarin's brow that wings upward and outward, exaggerating the line of the natural brow or totally obliterating it.

In its own way, the male eyebrow can make just as strong a statement as its female counterpart.

LEFT: *The Rock*

BELOW: *John L. Lewis*

OPPOSITE TOP: *Divine*

OPPOSITE BOTTOM: *Michael Cameron Benbrook, RuPaul, Lypsinka*

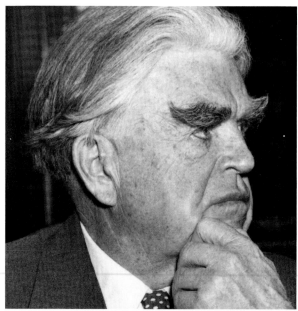

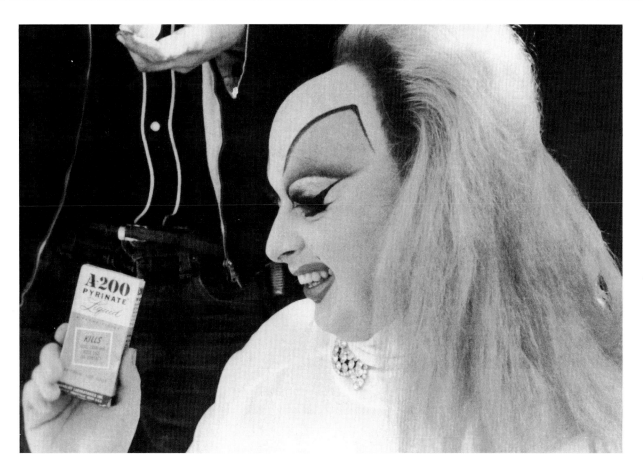

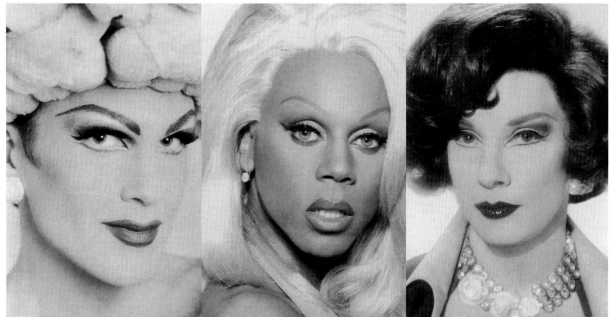

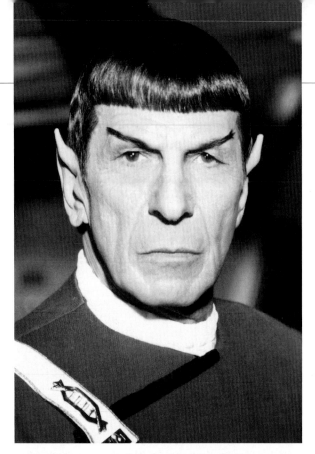

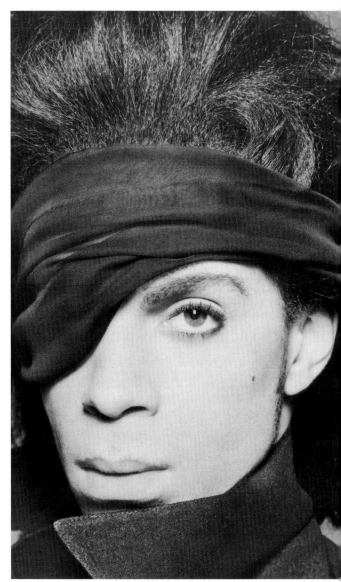

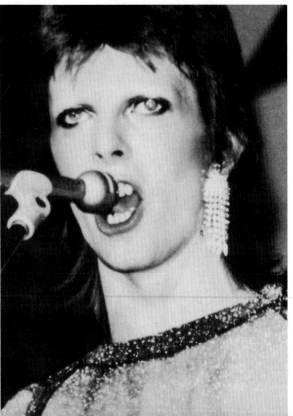

TOP LEFT: *Leonard Nimoy as Mr. Spock*

LEFT: *David Bowie*

ABOVE: *The Artist Formerly Known as Prince*

OPPOSITE: *José Manuel Carreño*

OPPOSITE RIGHT, TOP TO BOTTOM: *Yuri Grigoriev, Leonide Massine, Rudolf Nureyev*

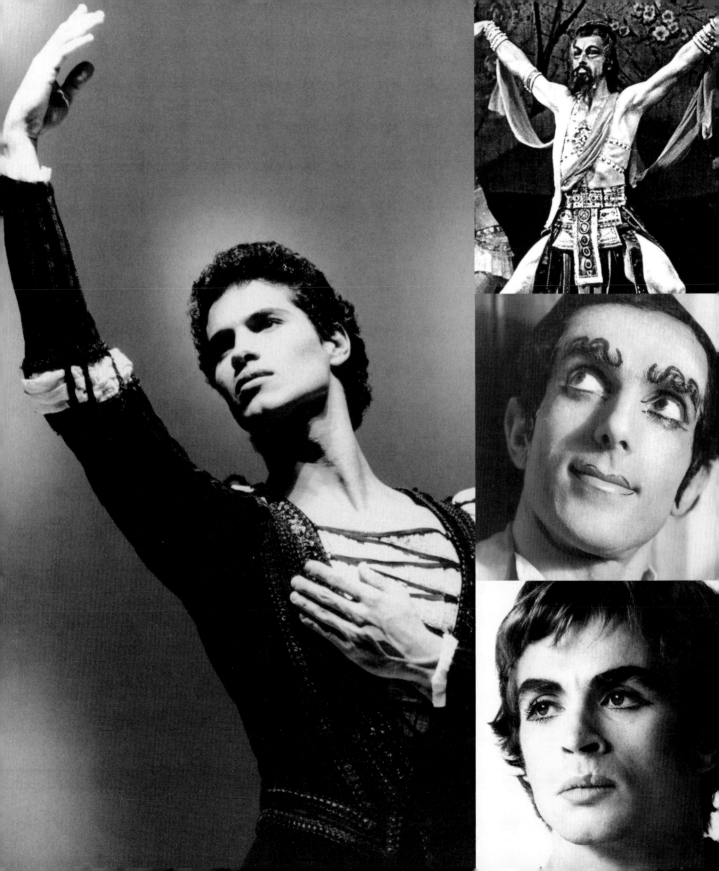

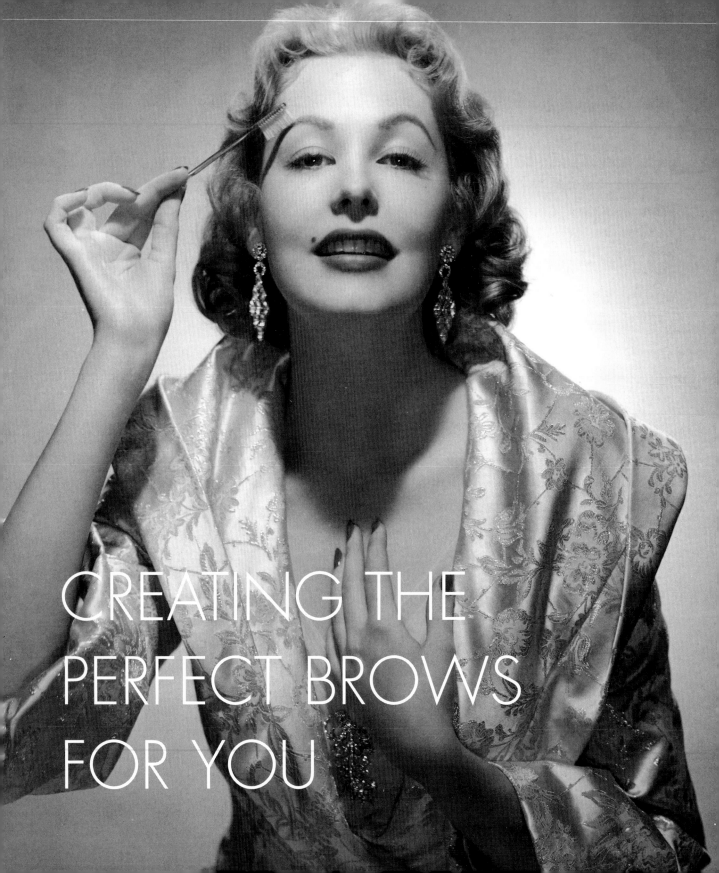

CREATING THE
PERFECT BROWS
FOR YOU

would love it if every one of you could sit in my chair, or at least have a professional makeup artist or esthetician examine and groom your eyebrows. There are, however, a few factors that could prevent it.

First of all, availability of a qualified and practiced makeup artist whose eye and hand can create the perfect brow on you. Second, the time factor. Although once you're sitting in the chair of a professional, the process itself isn't all that long (my clients, on average, are there for five, ten minutes maximum), getting there may be difficult.

There is also the money factor. Once you've had your eyebrows groomed by a specialist, you must maintain them. I have always recommended that my clients see me once a month. Many women, however, can afford neither the time nor the money.

This chapter is devoted to those of you who for any number of valid reasons would rather do it yourselves. Although, if possible, before you even start, you should try to visit a makeup artist or an esthetician who is very familiar with the process of setting a line. There are a few ways you can find a person to help establish your browline. Your hairdresser may have a suggestion, photographers who specialize in glamour portraits always know accomplished makeup artists, or you could visit a local day spa that specializes in facials and eyebrow care and ask for their recommendations.

Grooming your own brows is not difficult, although it may seem as daunting as performing surgery on yourself. All it requires is patience, an objective eye, and a steady hand. So, let us begin.

WHAT KIND OF BROWS DO I HAVE?

Before doing your own brows, it is absolutely necessary to figure out how your brow should be shaped for your particular face, eyes, and bone structure. I am not a trend person. If brows are looking sparse, shiny, or anemic on the fashion runway simply because a designer has decreed that they will be so for the next fifteen minutes, I ignore it.

As I mentioned earlier, at one time makeup artist Kevyn Aucoin advocated tinting brows lighter than your natural hair color. And a few years ago, New York designer Todd Oldham pasted graphic, thick, black fake eyebrows on his runway models, setting off chatter in fashion magazines that a trend toward heavier, darker brows was coming. But my skill has always been designing a brow specifically for the face of the client who is in my chair. It is something you can learn to do for yourself.

Before we start, let's try an exercise.

Sit in your chair near excellent natural light and hold a plain hand mirror in front of your face to get the big picture. I always recommend a hand mirror to begin because you can hold it as close to you as possible, and you won't have the barrier of your bathroom sink between you and your mirror.

Be very objective here. Analyze your brows. Are

they heavy? Are they light? Do they have a natural arch in them? Do they sit on your brow bone with no arch? Do they march across your nose? Are the hairs in your eyebrows thick and plentiful, or are they sparse and thin? Do these hairs slant? Do they curl? Are they short? Is one eyebrow thicker than the other? Do your eyes look too close together? Do your brows make your expression look angry?

How your brows are shaped can change your appearance. An example: One of my clients once told me, "My eyebrows betray my innermost emotions."

"Why?" I asked.

"Because," she said, "everyone says I look so angry." She had a very small face and extremely heavy brows that sat much too close together. I took out the heaviness near her nose, found her arch, and removed the hairs that obscured it. The result: Her new eyebrows opened up her face. She looked more relaxed because her brows did not appear furrowed in anxiety or anger.

Another woman told me when I cleaned up the hairs under her brows, "You've given me an instant face lift." And still another said that she looked as if she'd lost weight when I took out most of her heavy brow.

So, it is possible to change your whole look with judicious tweezing. Who knows what might happen? Changing the shape of a brow has changed the course of a career. For example, take actress Teri Hatcher (who played Superman's girlfriend, Lois Lane, on television). When she first started out, her eyebrows were heavy and rather thick. They gave her face a naive, innocent look, and her Girl-Next-Door roles reflected that. Then a makeup artist shaped her brow, made it narrower, discovered her gorgeous, expressive arch, and gave Hatcher a more worldly, sexy look. She went from everybody's nonthreatening best friend to Bombshell with a flick of the tweezer.

Perhaps no one of our current crop of superstars has changed her brows (and the rest of her look) as much as Madonna. When she first started out, her brows were thick and ungroomed, and matched her natural dark hair color. As she became more and more sophisticated as a performer, her brows were manicured. Narrowed. Lightened. Until there were hardly any brows left at all. Every time she changed her persona, she changed her look—from street urchin to Blond Bombshell, soignée siren to brooding Goth sorceress, new mother to New Age princess. For every new look, her eyebrows have gone through radical transformations.

THE THICK AND THIN OF IT

How thin should you make your brows?
Thin is not a look for everyone. It gives the face a severe appearance and requires constant supervision and maintenance. Not everyone can have a personal makeup artist at their beck and call the way 1920s film stars Jean Harlow and Clara Bow could, when their brows were mere wisps of pencil and shine. If your face and your personal style are complimented

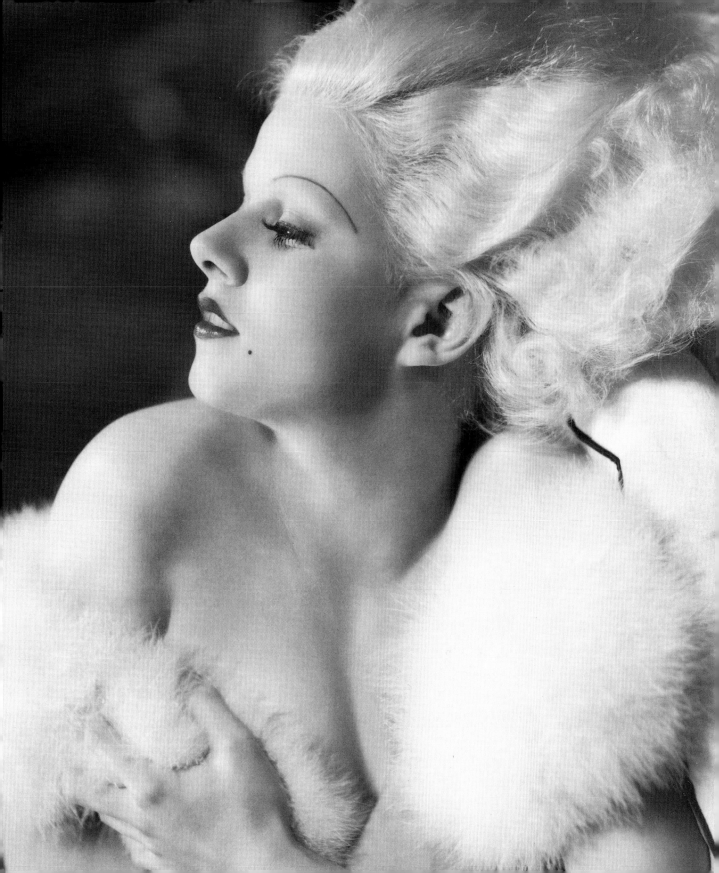

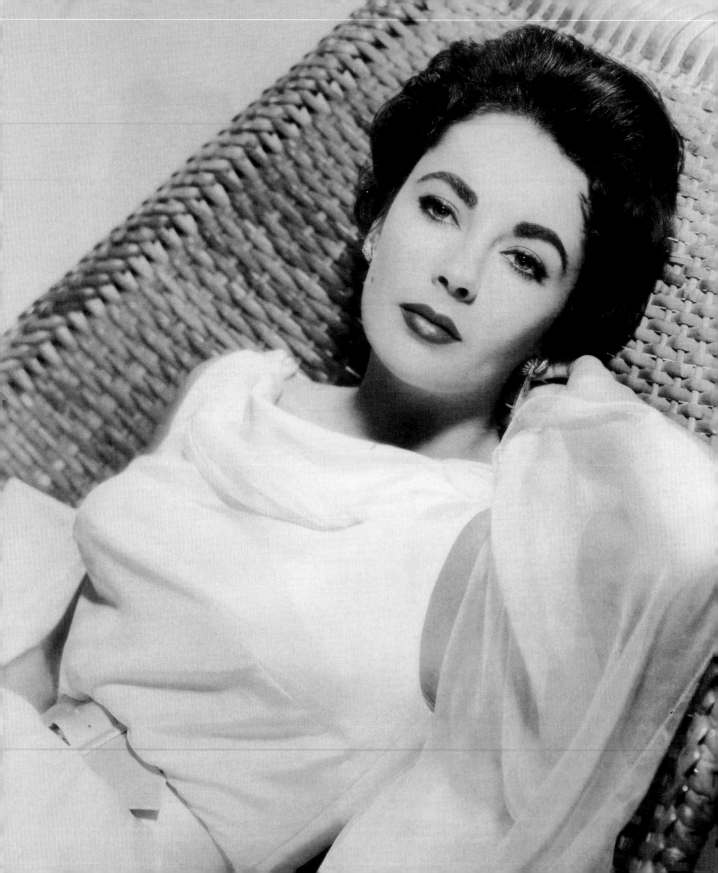

by a retro look, you can compare yourself favorably with a silent film star, and if you are reasonably young, then go for it. But remember, the skinnie-minnie brow is not only dated, it can make the face appear harsh, severe, and *old*.

A thin brow requires constant maintenance. To keep it pristine and neat, you are going to have to live in front of your mirror, tweezers in hand.

Thick eyebrows can be gorgeous (think Audrey Hepburn, Brooke Shields, Elizabeth Taylor) as long as they aren't so overpowering that they're all anyone sees when they look at you.

If you've been blessed with a healthy, full head of hair, it's likely that your brows are thick and perhaps bushy. Thick hair and thick brows are not, however, the best combination. They can be too overwhelming. Something is going to have to go, and it's usually the size of the eyebrow. With thick brows, you want to define, refine, clean, streamline, and maintain the line. Neatness counts when you have a surfeit of hair.

By now, you've probably gotten the idea that no two eyebrows are alike. They vary from person to person. They can even vary on your own face, with one brow thicker than the other; one brow higher than the other, or one brow beautifully arched and the other, not so great.

Since it's difficult to look objectively at our own faces, the way we perceive our brows may not be completely accurate. As a reality check, it might be beneficial to ask a friend to give you some constructive criticism, such as, you haven't taken out

enough. Or, heaven forbid, you've taken out too much!

Which brings up a point: What if you make a mistake? What if you have removed hairs that are essential to the proper arch for your face? What if you've taken out too many hairs near your nose, so that your eyebrows appear truncated and too far apart? What if you've shaped your brows into a globular head and a teensy tail, like a chubby tadpole? And what if you've tweezed the ends of your brows off when trying to get them to come out even?

When you tweeze your own brows, you must develop patience. Perhaps on your first foray into creative tweezing, you've not removed enough, or you've taken two hairs at a time and left a small hole, or you've tweezed away so much that your brows are now too thin. Consider your brows like teensy bangs that a hairdresser has cut too short. Eventually they will grow out. It becomes a waiting game. Unfortunately, there is no "hair food" like Miracle-Gro to stimulate your brows into regrowing hair overnight.

There have been times, also, when the trend toward ultrathin brows caused women all over America to shave or tweeze their brows; in some instances, they never grew back. As we know, a lot of our older aunts, mothers, and grandmothers who wanted the same sophisticated look as Jean Harlow shaved their eyebrows off and found to their dismay that they would not grow back. (Conversely, Brooke Shields started a trend toward thicker, more natural brows. So it does work both ways.)

Elizabeth Taylor

I learned to have patience when I made huge changes in my eyebrows when I was a teenager. I was one of the lucky ones when, in my hippie days, I took a razor to my thick brows. Fortunately, when my temporary madness passed, the brows grew back in, as thick and luxuriant as before. But I think it was back then, as I waited for each hair to reappear, that I first realized that trends may last for a few months, but eyebrows, really good ones, can last for life.

GETTING STARTED: THE RIGHT STUFF

Before you take tweezers to your brows and attempt to pull out the first hair, you have to have the right equipment. Don't be afraid to spend some money on a first-rate pair of stainless steel tweezers. Unless you lose them, a fine pair of tweezers can last a very long time. You should, however, have them sharpened by the manufacturer (if possible) or by a cutlery store when they dull. My favorite is the flat-slant or mitered-edge tweezer, which makes it easier for a nonprofessional to grab a hair. If not used expertly, pointed tweezers can pinch or poke your skin.

Excellent tweezers have good tension, which means that you can't close them very easily. They must also feel at home in your fingers. Size-wise, however, it's all a matter of personal taste, of what feels comfortable to you. Other necessary tools include a magnifying mirror, a combination eyebrow brush/comb, and a small pair of straight-edged scissors (not curved manicure scissors). Extras that might help you are a brow powder that matches the

172

base color of your hair; a semistiff-bristled, flat-edge brush; a regular lead pencil; and a white pencil.

It's always best to use a magnifying mirror when you do your brows yourself. Make sure that you can see exactly what you're working on, close up, when you choose a mirror. You might want to get an illuminated makeup mirror that you can install right in your bathroom and pull close to you, or use a portable with two separate sides—one for magnification and the other so that as you are working you can assess your brows in relationship to your eyes and the rest of your face.

Thus equipped, it's time to begin. But there are a few things you should do before you pick up your tweezers and start to pull out hairs.

TRIMMING YOUR BROWS

Your brows may have wild hairs that need to be trimmed. To find them, take your eyebrow comb

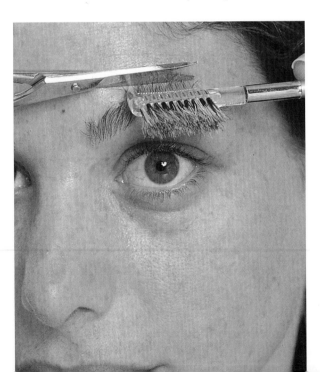

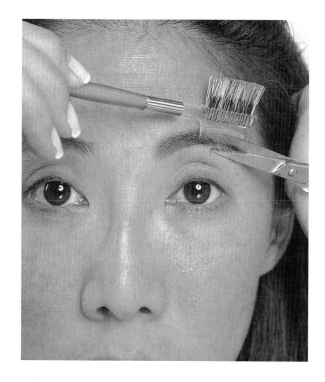

and groom your brows, brushing upward and then in the direction of your temples, the right side going right and the left side to the left. That way, you can see if there are any hairs that refuse to grow the way they should.

What do you do with a wild hair? If it is really curly and has a mind of its own, lift it upward

LEFT: *Lisa trimming. Lift the hairs upward with a brow comb and trim off any hairs that extend beyond the edge of the comb with a small, sharp scissors . . . carefully, please.*

ABOVE: *Cathy trimming. Be sure to comb hairs in the direction of growth before trimming.*

with a brow comb and trim it off with your small, straight-edged scissors. Be careful to trim only one hair at a time, and err on the conservative side. You don't want to give your eyebrows an instant crew cut.

Check the natural direction of hair growth. If your eyebrows grow downward, be sure to brush them downward and trim across the bottom.

THE PENCIL TRICK

Now comes the fun part: discovering the perfect brows for your face.

The keys to beautiful brows are to eliminate the negative and intensify the positive. One of the best ways to begin is simply to draw on the brow you think you'd like using an eyebrow powder that most matches your natural brow color, imagining what it would look like if the hairs that didn't fit your ideal brow weren't there.

There is a very precise method that I call the Pencil Trick that will help you find where to draw on your perfect fantasy brow before you even remove the first hair. First, consider beginnings and endings.

Step One
How far should the perfect brow extend in either direction? The perfect brow ideally begins just above the inside corner of your eye. To find that point exactly, take a pencil, an orange stick, or a small ruler and hold it perpendicular from the side of your nose

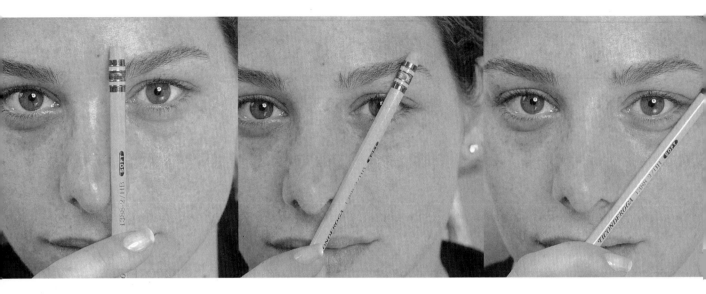

to your eyebrow. Where brow and pencil meet is where your eyebrow should begin.

Step Two

Remember that the shape of your naturally beautiful brow should always follow the curve of the eye. The arch of the brow achieves its highest point directly above the iris, or colored part of your eye. To find that place, lay your pencil again diagonally from the center of your bottom lip, past the edge of your nose, and slant it to the outside corner of the iris. Your arch is at the *inside* edge of the pencil where it meets the brow.

Step Three

To determine where your brow should stop, place your pencil in the center of your lip, slanting it on an angle to the outside edge of the eye. Your brow should end at the *inside* edge of the pencil.

I'm sure you've met women who didn't know when to stop drawing their eyebrows. They may have extended them far past the edge of the eye, and perhaps downward like a very large comma. The effect makes them look sad or dissatisfied. What you are trying to achieve is *balance:* eyebrows that don't start so far over toward your nose that they appear to bring your eyes too close together and that don't extend so far that you look sad, scared, or angry.

Now, dip a small, flat-bristled, angled brush in brow powder and, using tiny, upward movements as if you're drawing on one hair at a time, lightly sketch in your ideal eyebrow. Then take a white pencil and "erase" the extra hairs. Using the non-magnification side of your mirror, look at your reflection and judge what you've done in concert with the rest of your face.

TIME TO TWEEZE

So, you've analyzed your brows, trimmed the wild hairs, drawn on your ideal eyebrow, and blocked out the hairs that don't belong with concealer pencil. Now, seat yourself comfortably, preferably at a table with a mirror on it and near a source of natural light, which always works best. Be sure your hands and tools are clean before you begin. To be absolutely sure you're working with clean instruments, sterilize your tweezers with alcohol or very hot water and wash your hands in antibacterial soap.

If you are sensitive to tweezing, you might also

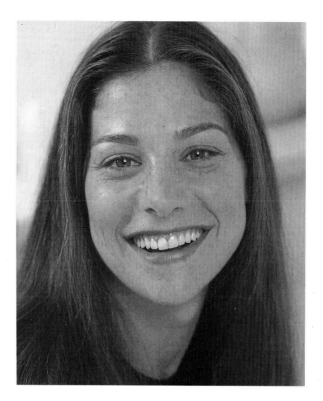

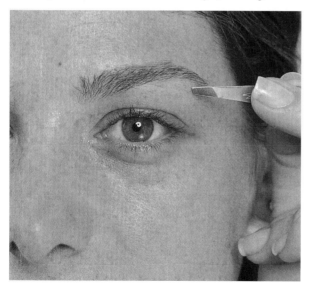

want to "prime" the area you'll be working on. You can numb the brow first with an ice cube, or if you want to make things easier on yourself, you can soak a cloth or cotton balls in hot water, wring the cloth out, and press it on the brow area for a few seconds to open up the hair follicles. (If you've wiped off any brow pencil and concealer, you might want to reapply them before you tweeze.)

LEFT: *Lisa tweezing. Carefully tweeze one brow at a time, pulling the hair out in the direction that it grows.*

ABOVE: *Lisa after.*

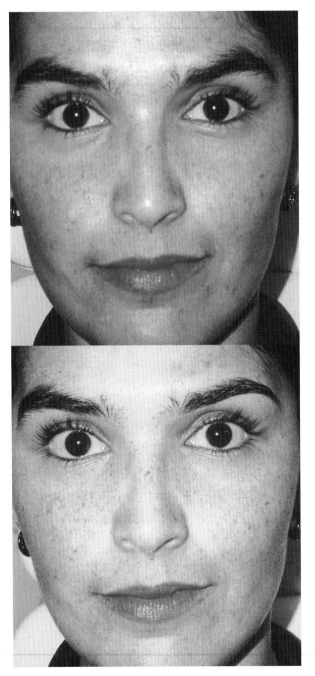

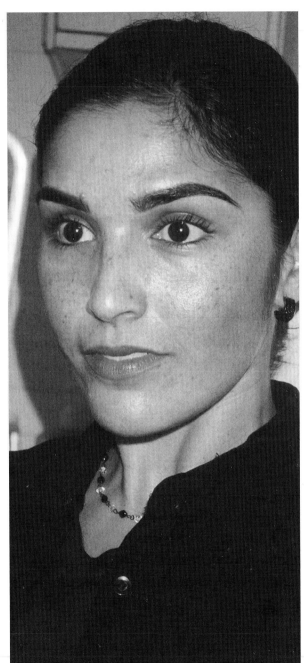

Be sure that as you tweeze, you are pulling unwanted hair out in the direction it grows, which is toward the ear. The hairs will come out easier, and it will probably hurt less. Be sure to pull hairs out one at a time, not in clumps or bunches, because you might take too much and leave holes that will take several weeks to grow back in.

Simply remove the extra hairs that do not conform to your ideal eyebrow. Some people alternate tweezing eyebrows, removing a hair from one and then a corresponding hair from the other. I prefer to do one brow at a time. Remember, your face is not symmetrical, and neither are your eyebrows. Finish one and then start the other, trying to get it to look as much like the finished brow as possible.

Don't be afraid to remove extra hairs on top of your natural brow. Our mothers may have told us never to tweeze on the top, but it is sometimes necessary in order to keep a clean line. Just don't go near the essence of the brow itself, where you've drawn on your perfect brow.

When you're done, you'll probably notice that where you've removed the stray hairs, your skin may be red and the area may be a little puffy. This will go away shortly. To eliminate the irritation, put some

TOP LEFT: *Diana has such thick brows that there's plenty of room to find her ideal brow.*

BOTTOM LEFT: *Diana with one brow groomed.*

LEFT: *Diana, after.*

ice in a bowl of water and soak a clean washcloth. Wring it out and gently hold the cloth on your brow. Another instant soother: cotton balls soaked in witch hazel. If, however, your eyebrow area begins to itch or you develop a rash or bumps, use an over-the-counter cortisone cream to ease your discomfort. Fresh aloe is another excellent anti-irritant. If you have an aloe plant, break off a leaf and use nature's own calmative directly on the redness.

To finish your brows, use a brow gel or a clear mascara or even a bit of hairspray on your eyebrow brush and brush your brows upward and outward in the direction the hairs grow, to display them to their full effect.

DEALING WITH LIGHT-COLORED OR SPARSE BROWS

Women with very light-colored skin and hair and women with sparse eyebrows have their own specific problems. There are a few tricks of the trade that can make grooming your brows a lot easier.

If you have blond hair and a light complexion, chances are your brows are either too light to register, have a lot of gray hairs, or barely exist at all. They need help.

The brush-and-powder method of filling in the brows before you tweeze is also an excellent first step for women with very light brows. You can fill them in with a small, flat, angled brush dipped in a brow powder that is the base color of your hair or slightly darker.

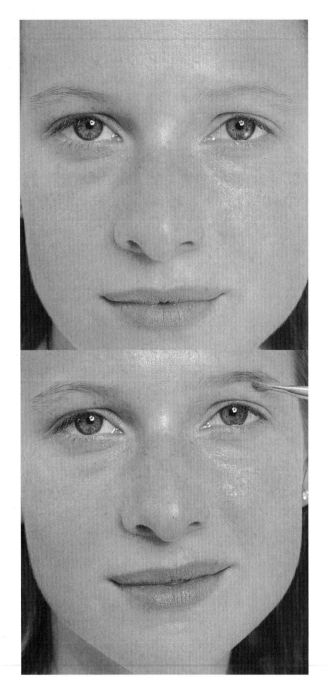

Dip the brush into the powder gently and blow off the excess (you can also remove the excess by tapping the brush on the edge of your hand or the sink) and lightly, very lightly, fill in your brows with the color. If you've put too much color on the brush, test the amount on the back of your hand and remove the excess before you sketch in your brows.

Use a very light touch. The effect you want is as close to nature as possible. Remember, less is best. Brow powder needs to appear delicately applied, like the gossamer brush strokes in a Japanese painting. Don't glop it on or draw a harsh, single line. We're not going for the drag queen, *Mommie Dearest* look.

Now, tweeze the "negative"—the hairs that aren't within the brow you've drawn with powder.

Once you've created your ideal shape, define your brows with tinted gel. How dark should a blonde make her eyebrows? That is completely a matter of taste. While I recommend matching the

TOP: *Light, sparse brows need help: Christy, before.*

BOTTOM: *Filling in: Christy uses brush and powder.*

RIGHT TOP: *Tweezing the negative and leaving the positive.*

RIGHT BOTTOM: *Defining with tinted brow gel.*

FAR RIGHT: *Christy, after.*

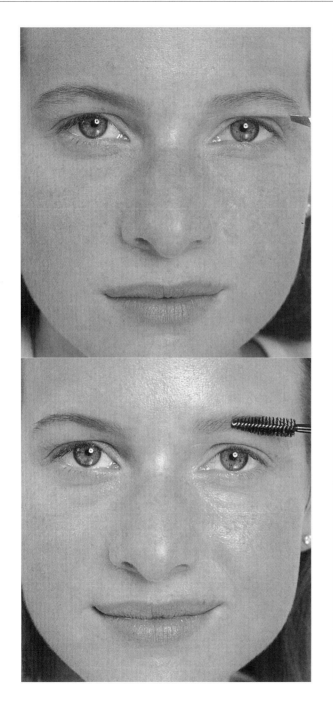

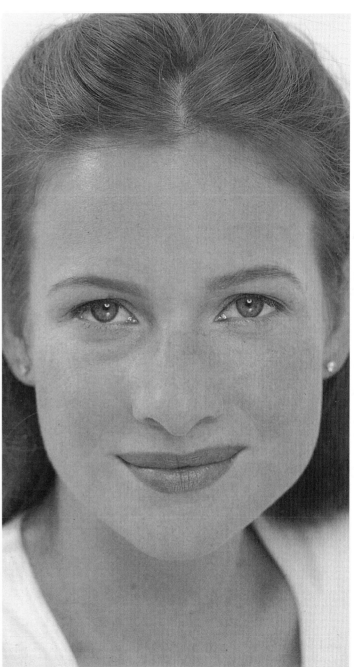

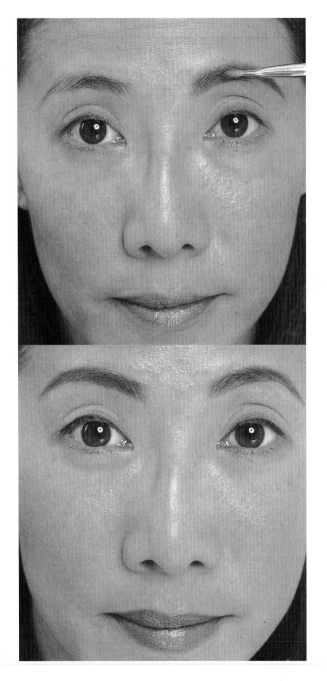

base color of the hair with a complementary brow powder to define a light brow, some blondes, like actress Sharon Stone, prefer (and look great) with relatively dark brows.

Even women with dark hair can have sparse brows that need filling in. As always, before you begin to determine the correct placement of your brow, you should use the powder-and-brush method to achieve the desired shape. Finish with tinted brow gel for dramatic definition.

What if you have only a very few hairs, or no eyebrows at all? Perhaps you tweezed overzealously at one time, and now the brows won't grow back. Or perhaps you've gone through menopause and lost hormones, including estrogen and testosterone, that affect hair growth. As women grow older, they lose body hair. Sometimes they don't have to shave their legs or under their arms very often, if at all. And sometimes the hair on their head and eyebrows thins. Also, if a woman undergoes chemotherapy treatment for cancer, she may lose her hair.

If you're really creating your eyebrows from scratch, you may want to use eye shadow powder, applied with a tiny brush (pencils tend to be greasy and produce an unnatural shine on the brow bone). Or you may want to consider tattooing, although it may be a permanent solution to a temporary prob-

TOP: *Cathy fills in her brow with powder.*
BOTTOM: *Cathy, after.*

TOP: *Wanata's eyebrows register very faintly on her skin.*

BOTTOM: *Wanata, after. She fills her brows in with a medium black eyebrow powder, then tweezes out the superfluous hairs.*

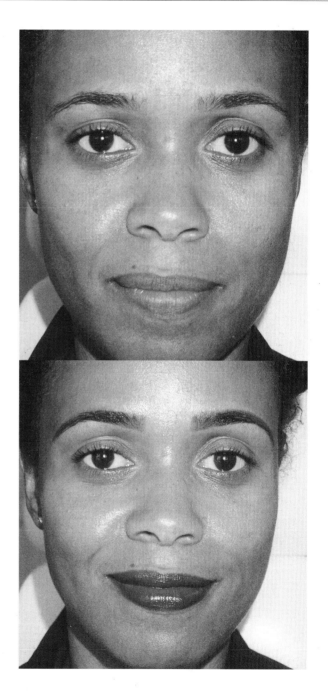

lem, and I wouldn't do it unless I knew the tattoo artist was really excellent. The only person in Los Angeles that I trust to tattoo my clients is Sheila May. She is skilled at drawing patterns of hair with very real-looking fine lines. Since not everyone can come to Los Angeles for Sheila's marvelous art, I recommend finding a tattooist who has a very light, artistic touch and asking to see photographs of his or her work.

BROW MAINTENANCE

You've trimmed and tweezed your brows and gotten them (almost) where you want them. (Don't be discouraged, by the way, if your brows don't look perfect the first time. When I'm working with a new client, it might take a few visits to get her brows into beautiful shape. You must have patience.)

Now, it's the next day. Your face is clean, you look at your handiwork in your bathroom mirror, and you realize that your brows are not even. The easiest thing to do is to fill them in with brow powder with your small mitered-edge brush. Set the powder with brow gel.

When you get the hang of it, doing your brows

181

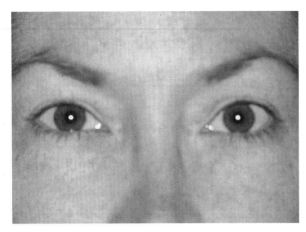

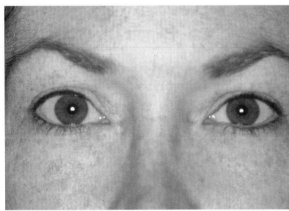

Gina, before and after tattooing.

yourself will become easier and easier. Once you've gotten your brows where you want them, maintenance is a snap because you're only going after stray hairs. Examine your brows once or twice a week and tweeze out any hairs that have grown back. Keep up with it, and you won't have to perform a major excavation job ever again.

THE FINAL CHECKLIST: DOS AND DON'TS

Do

- Plan first, before you tweeze.
- Use excellent light; natural light is preferable.
- Keep your hands and your equipment clean.
- Take only the hairs that are the "negative."
- For finishing touches, use brow powder, not pencil.
- Use finishing gel: either brow groomer or transparent mascara.

Don't

- Never tweeze without a plan. Make your ideal shape first with powder and concealer.
- Never tweeze into the basic eyebrow itself. Take only the stray hairs.
- Avoid eyebrow pencils. They contain wax and can look fake and obvious.
- Don't remove more than one hair at a time.
- Keep your fingers off the freshly tweezed area if they are not absolutely clean.

I cannot emphasize this enough: Balance is the key. The eyebrow is your face's frame. When you have a great brow, you don't need a lot of makeup.

Finally, here are the two most important points to remember: Have patience, and practice makes perfect. Good luck!

Mae West

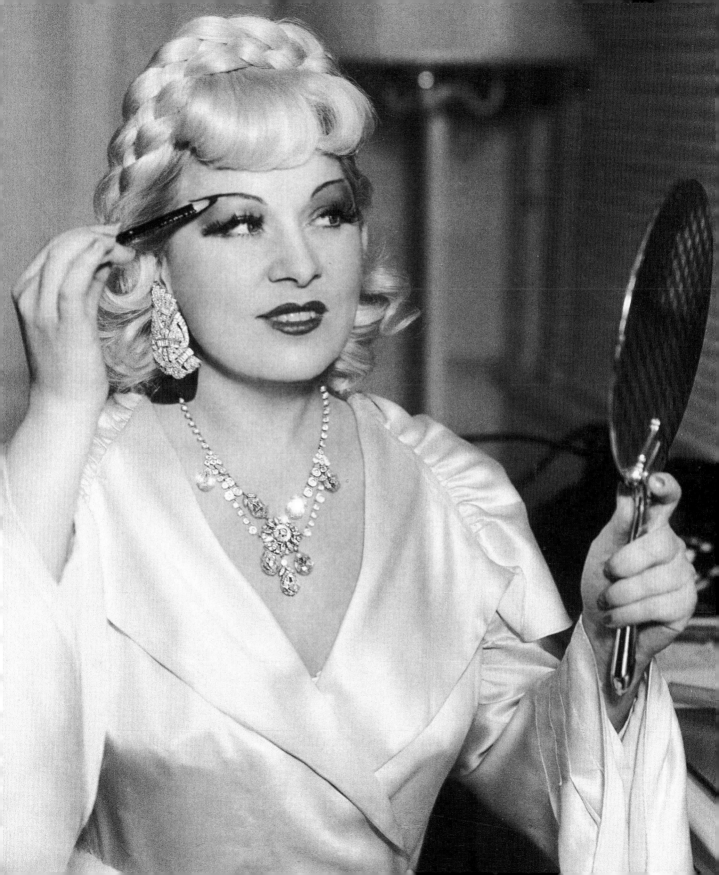

ACKNOWLEDGMENTS

Much love and gratitude to the following people:

My dear mom—I bet when I came out of the bathroom in 1965 with both of my eyebrows completely shaved off, you never would have believed in a million years that I would write a book on the subject! My wonderful dad—who gave me my love of art and beauty. My sister, Wendy—I just don't know what I would have done without your help, artistic and otherwise. Who would have thought that through this project we would find the meaning of true sisterhood? A special thank-you to my entire family: Uncle Nate and Molly, for being so supportive of me. Aunt Rose, for still having time for me, with all that you've been through this past year. You're amazing! Aunt Ida, for giving me my very first introduction to the eyebrow. I was mesmerized as I watched you tweeze them out night after night, hair after hair, in front of your vanity mirror, and now they're all gone!

Irit Ehrlich, for always being there every step of the way—not just for this book, but for my life. Debra Lynn Jones, for always listening and making my big problems seem small again. Your logic balances me out. Marsha Harris, my oldest friend, for helping me immensely with the selection of photographs—and with everything else through the years. My great friend Zina Chernus, for always yelling at me when needed and trying to keep me on the straight and narrow. Bonnie Vogel, for your constant support, love, and suggestions. Jac Dubelle and Louis Dell'Olio, for your love, support, and great friendship. Wanata Parker, for a midnight talk every night. You help me decompress with your down-home wisdom. Jym Genesta, for always being there to blow out my hair at the last minute and for being so generous with everything. Terry Ongaro, who is always there through all the laughter and tears. You're my steel magnolia. Jean Jacques Cesbron and Paula Parisot, for your enthusiasm about my project and your help with photo selection.

Trevor Enoch, the very first person to help me in my very first selection of photographs for this book. Ken Chernus—you always make everyone look great with your incredible photography. You're a wonderful friend. Veronica Hinman, beauty director at *Glamour,* for so much help and support. Joel Freeman, for all your great advice and wonderful words of support.

Amy Pascal, for allowing me access to your extensive film library in your movie kingdom, Columbia Studios. Leslie Brill, creative executive at Columbia Studios, for always being there any time, any day for proper guidance, great information, and terrific leads. The late Dawn Steel, for teaching me how even to begin this project. ("It's called f——ing research, Robyn!")

My friends at the Peter Coppola Salon in New York City, with special thanks to Rudy Sprogis, Erin Sartain, Luis Mora, and Ronda Conley for always supporting me and being so helpful in times of stress, and also Steven Amendola, Hervé Bauge, Tony Flanders, Burton Machen, Kevin Mancuso, Dana

Nicosia, and Wayne Nishyama. Special thanks to Jason "A" Low, for our important meetings on the stairs. Sweet Ivette Rodriguez, for all your assistance. All the editors at the magazines and newspapers that have supported my career in makeup and eyebrows through the years: *Allure, Details, Detour, Elle, Glamour, Good Housekeeping, Harper's Bazaar, InStyle, Jane, Ladies' Home Journal, Latina,* the *Los Angeles Times, Mademoiselle, Marie Claire, Mirabella, Mode,* the *New York Times, Vogue,* and *W.* The great production staff and beautiful dancers of the American Ballet Theatre, for your encouragement and support, especially José Manuel Carreño, Julie Kent, Keith Roberts, Angel Corella, Giray Atalay, Rosalie O'Conner, David Richardson, Donya Hubby, and Lori Rosecrans.

Rebecca Rubin Akhan, administrative assistant to the Black & White Photo Library at the Metropolitan Museum of Art; James Kilvington in the rights and reproductions department of the Picture Library at the National Portrait Gallery in London; Jacklyn Burns, rights and reproductions coordinator in the photo services department at the J. Paul Getty Museum; and Kimberly Gilhooly, rights and reproductions at the Norton Simon Museum. Thanks to all of you for assisting me with my research and granting permission to use all the beautiful art images. Michael Stier, senior permissions coordinator at *Vogue* / Condé Nast publications, for his kindness and patience, and his help with all my fashion photograph dilemmas. Ron and Howard Mandelbaum at Photofest for allowing me to do a large portion of my photo research in their wonderful archives. Marc Wanamaker, film and Los Angeles city historian, for being so generous with his time, his vast knowledge of Hollywood history, and his beautiful photographs. Daniel Nicoletta, for his fascinating photographs.

Christy Beck, Lisa Tarlow, Cathy Yamasaki, Diana Romo, and Wanata Parker for their patience in sitting for the "how to" chapter. Thanks, girls! Sheila May for allowing me to use her before-and-after photographs of tattooed eyebrows. A special thank-you to Cynthia Robins, for your genius in writing and knowing how to bring me out onto these pages. You're not only great, you're fast! Judith Regan, the best in the business. I have great respect and admiration for you, not only as a publisher but as a woman. Thank you for believing in me. Cassie Jones—I don't know what I would do if I did not talk to you ten times a day! You are a great editor and made the hard stuff much easier—and fun, too. Renée Iwaszkiewicz, for your good cheer and invaluable help in pulling the whole book together. Art directors Jeannette Jacobs, Charles Rue Woods, and Joseph Montebello for making this book look so beautiful. Justin Whitman, for all your work and support.

Finally, special thanks to all my clients on both coasts for your loyalty, even when I yell, "Leave them alone! Do not touch!"

BIBLIOGRAPHY

Angeloglou, Maggie. *A History of Makeup*. Great Britain: Macmillan, 1970.

Basten, Fred E., and Paul A. Kaufman. *Max Factor's Hollywood, Glamour, Movies, Make-Up*. Los Angeles: General Publishing Group, 1995.

Batterberry, Michael and Ariane. *Mirror Mirror: A Social History of Fashion*. New York: Holt, Rinehart, and Winston, 1977.

Corson, Richard. *Fashion in Makeup, from Ancient to Modern Times*. New York: Universe Books, 1972.

Daniel, Clifton, editor. *Chronicle of the Twentieth Century*. Mt. Kisco, New York: Chronicle Publications, 1987.

De Castlebajac, Kate. *The Face of the Century: 100 Years of Makeup and Style*. New York: Rizzoli, 1995.

Donavan, Hedley, editor. *Life Goes to the Movies*. New York: *Time*, 1975.

Eames, John Douglas. *The MGM Story*. New York: Crown, 1977.

Garland, Madge. *The Changing Face of Beauty: Four Thousand Years of Beautiful Women*. New York: Barrows and Company, 1957.

Larkin, Rochelle. *Hail, Columbia*. New Rochelle, New York: Arlington House Publishers, 1975.

Maltin, Leonard. *Leonard Maltin's 1999 Movie and Video Guide*. New York: Plume, 1998.

Manvell, Dr. Roger, editor. *The International Encyclopedia of Film*. New York: Crown, 1972.

Miller, Jean-Chris. *The Body Art Book: A Complete, Illustrated Guide to Tattoos, Piercings, and Other Body Modifications*. New York: Berkley Books, 1997.

Moffitt, Peggy, and William Claxton. *The Rudi Gernreich Book*. Köln, Germany: Taschen, 1999.

Mulvey, Kate, and Melissa Richards. *Decades of Beauty: The Changing Image of Women, 1890s to 1990s*. New York: Checkmark Books, 1998.

Potterton, David, editor. *Culpeper's Color Herbal*. New York: Sterling Publishing, 1983.

Sennett, Ted. *Hollywood Musicals*. New York: Harry N. Abrams, 1981.

Shipman, David. *The Great Movie Stars: The Golden Years*. New York: Hill and Wang, 1970.

CREDITS

Bison Archives: pages 30, 33, 40, 51, 53 bottom, 72, 91 right.

Peter C. Borsari Photography: page xiv.

Ken Chernus: pages v, xvii, xviii, 172–75, 178, 180.

Courtesy Robyn Cosio: first photo in contents, pages x, xi, xii left, xiii, xv, 176, 181.

Robert Crikman: page 165 left.

Arthur Elgort: eighth photo in contents; page 147.

J. Paul Getty Museum: pages 5, 18.

Courtesy Yuri Grigoriev: page 165 top right.

George Holz: page 140.

Sheila May: page 182.

Metropolitan Museum of Art: second photo in contents; pages xx, 3, 12, 14, 20, 22.

National Portrait Gallery, London: page 8.

Daniel Nicoletta: pages 146, 163 bottom left, 163 bottom right (hair by Deena Davenport, make-up by Patrick Toomy).

Norton Simon Museum: page 7.

Rosalie O'Conner, Corps de Ballet, American Ballet Theatre: page 143.

Photofest: pages ii–iii (Hedy Lamarr); third through sixth photos in contents; pages viii, 24, 26, 29, 34, 36, 39, 41–50, 52, 53 top, 54–56, 58, 60–71, 74, 78, 82–90, 91 left, 92–98, 100–105, 107–12, 114, 115, 118–20, 122–32, 134, 136, 139, 141, 142, 144, 148–61, 162 right, 163 bottom center, 164, 165 right center and right bottom, 166, 168, 170, 183.

Matthew Rolston: seventh photo in contents (Judith Regan).

Richard Vogel: page xii right.

Vogue/Condé Nast publications: pages
75 left (Condé Nast Archive),
75 right and 81 (Erwin Blumenfeld),
76 (René R. Bouché),
77 (Richard Rutledge),
79 (Karen Radkai),
80 (William Bell),
106 (Franco Rubartelli),
116 (Chris Von Wangenheim),
117 (Francesco Scavullo),
135 (Peter Lindbergh),
137 (Arthur Elgort),
138 (Dewey Nicks).

World Wrestling Federation Entertainment, Inc.: page 162 left.

About the Authors

ROBYN COSIO is a well-known makeup artist in Los Angeles and New York City who specializes in eyebrows. Her clients include Christina Applegate, Marisa Tomei, Gina Gershon, Jamie Lee Curtis, Laura San Giacomo, Vanessa Redgrave, Jennifer Grey, Jody Watley, Joan Chen, Lesley Stahl, and Elizabeth Perkins. She has been interviewed as an authority on eyebrows and makeup in *Vogue, InStyle, Bazaar, W, Elle, Marie Claire, Mademoiselle, Allure,* and many other magazines and on CNN, *Today,* FOX, and MTV and has designed makeup for Louis Dell'Olio and Donna Karan for Anne Klein, Calvin Klein, and Bill Blass. She lives in Beverly Hills, California.

Robyn has created an eyebrow kit to help you craft your own perfect eyebrows. For information: 1-877-EYE-BRWS or www.eleganteyebrow.com.

CYNTHIA ROBINS is the fashion and beauty editor of the *San Francisco Examiner* and the author of three books on fashion and beauty. She lives in San Francisco, California.